FOLLOWERSHIP

A Practical Guide

to Aligning Leaders

and Followers

FOLLOWERSHIP

A Practical Guide

to Aligning Leaders

and Followers

Tom Atchison

ACHE Management Series

Health Administration Press

Your board, staff, or clients may also benefit from this book's insight. For more information on quantity discounts, contact the Health Administration Press Marketing Manager at (312) 424-9470.

This publication is intended to provide accurate and authoritative information in regard to the subject matter covered. It is sold, or otherwise provided, with the understanding that the publisher is not engaged in rendering professional services. If professional advice or other expert assistance is required, the services of a competent professional should be sought.

The statements and opinions contained in this book are strictly those of the author and do not represent the official positions of the American College of Healthcare Executives or of the Foundation of the American College of Healthcare Executives.

08   07   06   05   04   5   4   3   2

Library of Congress Cataloging-in-Publication Data

Atchison, Thomas A., 1945–
     Followership : aligning leaders and followers / Tom Atchison.
        p. cm.
     Rev. ed. of: Turning health care leadership around / Thomas A. Atchison. 1st ed. 1990.
     Includes index.
     ISBN 1-56793-216-9 (alk. paper)
     1. Health services administrators—Psychology.   2. Health services
     administration—Psychological aspects.   3. Leadership—Psychological aspects.
     I. Atchison, Thomas A., 1945– Turning health care leadership around.   II. Title.

The paper used in this publication meets the minimum requirements of American National Standard for Information Sciences—Permanence of Paper for Printed Library Materials, ANSI Z39.48-1984. ∞TM

Acquisitions manager: Janet Davis; project manager: Joyce Sherman; cover design: Betsy Pérez

Health Administration Press
A division of the Foundation
    of the American College of
    Healthcare Executives
One North Franklin Street
Suite 1700
Chicago, IL 60606
(312) 424-2800

Contents

Preface

THIS BOOK IS a revision of my 1990 text on the role of leadership in healthcare. The title of that book is *Turning Healthcare Leadership Around*. When the American College of Healthcare Executives (ACHE) asked me to consider a revised edition of the book, I was not initially enthusiastic. However, I mentioned the revision proposal to my good friend Joe Bujak, with whom I coauthored a book on physician partnerships. Joe believed that the first book was still valid, except for the case material, and remarked that healthcare does not need yet another book on leadership. He suggested that I reframe the text as a guide for all healthcare professionals on the topic of "followership."

Joe is highly skilled at posing the "wicked" question and asked why an inverse relationship seems to exist between the number of books on leadership and the lack of effective leadership in healthcare. Current issues such as worsening morale and enduring staff shortages, results of psychologically toxic work environments, point to this lack. He recommended that I construct a text that looked at the dynamics of followers—that is, why someone would choose to align his or her interests to those of another person. What triggers followership? Joe's insight led me to rethink the opportunity for a revised text.

Another motivation, albeit a small motivator, for writing this book is that very few texts have been published on followership. A recent search of Amazon.com yielded a total of two related references. A search of *Harvard Business Review* resulted in only one short piece on the topic. Discussion of *followership* has not yet become mainstream, so this book represents an opportunity to share with you a comprehensive view of this very important notion. I hope you find it useful.

Tom Atchison
May 2003

Acknowledgments

THE PROCESS OF writing a book is a long, and sometimes lonely, journey. There may be authors who have the ability to walk this journey alone—I am not one of those people. This book was finished because of many people who played various roles, from cheerleaders to benign dictators. There was the main cheerleader: my dear wife Debbie. There were the wonderful people who did all the hard work: Letty and Elia. And there was the benign dictator: my good friend Julie.

I also want to thank the very helpful and supportive people at Health Administration Press: Audrey helped develop the book concept, and Janet did a great job of editing.

Finally, I wish to dedicate this book to my mother, Alice, who is the first real leader I experienced. She has lived a life of inspiring others to be the best they can be.

PART ONE

The New Leadership Mandate:
Followership

CHAPTER 1

Changing Healthcare Organizations: The Followership Difference

LEADERS HAVE FOLLOWERS. Being called the chief executive officer (CEO) and standing in front of a group does not in itself make anyone a leader. Without committed followers, you have nothing but a title. No matter how elegant your diversification strategy, how sophisticated the information systems, or how strong the financial base, you will never build an effective healthcare delivery system unless you can inspire others to follow.

Commitment to follow a leader results when the follower has transcended self-interest. Commitment is the glue that binds the followers to the leader. The most successful healthcare leaders are able to create this commitment from followers across all groups, including executives, managers, supervisors, physicians, and all other employees.

"Titled" healthcare executives can create new services, negotiate joint ventures, and build new alliances and still be little more than bean counters and management mechanics. It is in the behaviors and attitudes of their followers where we find the difference between titled executives and true leaders. Are you in the top position simply because someone hired you at a high salary level? If so, you are a titled executive, like the fabled "emperor" with "new clothes," not a leader. Leaders are in the top position because the staff follows them. Titled executives fix problems, whereas leaders inspire others to follow a vision. Followers want a leader who can articulate a vision of a better place than currently exists. Followers want to trust their leaders, they want hope and direction, and, most of all, they want recognition for achievement of successful results.

Healthcare leaders inspire followers to live the organization's mission and achieve its vision using the behaviors defined by its core values. The mission, values, and vision are more than rhetoric to a leader. Titled executives who just mouth the words *mission, values,* and *vision* cannot inspire followers. Through the force of their presence, leaders model the behaviors that inspire followers to become committed to the mission, achieve the vision, and live the values.

Today's healthcare environment makes the job of creating followers much more difficult and at the same time more important. The sense of disenfranchisement of healthcare workers continues to worsen because they are required to do more with less. Commiting to the mission, achieving the vision, and behaving according to the core values is thus increasingly difficult. Rebuilding commitment in one or more service areas of an organization seems to be constantly necessary, and the possibility of sustainable change and commitment seems to be very elusive in today's healthcare delivery environment. Long-term staff loyalty is now a rare phenomenon.

As healthcare executives struggle to find new ways to inspire followers, they represent the solutions as well as part of the problem. Bruised and battered by ever-changing expectations, many titled healthcare executives adopt rigid, autocratic management behaviors characterized by short-term thinking and supported by archaic myths about how to engage followers. If healthcare professionals are to inspire followers, they must reject these myths and counterproductive behaviors and create a corporate culture that nurtures followers.

What do noted healthcare executives Greg Carlson, CHE; William Foley, FACHE; Kelly Mather; and Kevin Nolan have in common? They all have committed followers. Throughout this book, you will see that although the organizations they head have different corporate structures, leadership styles, and markets, each one knows how to inspire staff to follow them. They understand that the intangible benefits and other factors that bring people into healthcare, such as caring for others, compassion, and the need to support and be supported, underpin much of the behavior seen in healthcare delivery systems. Although these healthcare leaders are different in many observable ways, they all possess the essential leadership traits of courage, energy, and discipline.

Carlson, Foley, Mather, and Nolan are recognized as true leaders because they build effective organizations by focusing on the people first and the programs second. All healthcare executives must now cope with rising expectations and decreasing net revenues as well as the accompanying increase in stress in their environments; the work environments in which these leaders inspire followers are no different. To avoid being caught in the undertow, leaders monitor the organization's pulse by interacting with employees. They create a corporate culture in which positive change can be sustained because the people who work in these cultures understand how they fit, they feel respected, and they are recognized for their contributions. However, creating a positive work environment that produces followers is not simple and takes time, rigor, and diligence. Success with this challenge hinges on the delicate and critical issues of values and meaning: Who are we, really? What are we doing here? Does anything we do matter? Are we making

> "For organizations to successfully adapt to the rapidly changing healthcare environment, leadership must author a compelling vision, identify the metrics that define success, communicate clear expectations, and hold individuals accountable for performance."
>
> —Joseph S. Bujak, M.D., vice president of medical affairs, Kootenai Medical Center, Coeur d'Alene, Idaho

a difference in people's lives? In short, followers want to work for healthcare executives who can answer these questions in a way that gives purpose to their efforts.

FROM COMPASSION TO CAPITALISM

Healthcare is an industry that no longer has a clear context. It was created to heal the sick; today, however, healthcare professionals are confused about what their job is. This confusion began in the mid-1980s when the industry's identity shifted from compassion to capitalism. "No margin, no mission" changed the focus of decision making from people to profit. The immensely toxic effect of this statement equated care to a profit or loss perspective. The resulting organizational impact is that employees (i.e., potential followers) are considered economic units. No employee will behave as a committed follower in a healthcare context that provides muddled or confusing messages about compassion and capital. Yet this is exactly the context in which healthcare executives must inspire staff to follow. Successful leaders are able to cut through the confusion by placing people, care, and service as the drivers of all decisions. To these leaders, money is only one metric of performance—it is not healthcare's *raison d'etre*.

All humans want meaning in their life. Very early we begin to learn to respond to stimuli as desirable or undesirable. We learn which environments are pleasant and recognize the characteristics of unpleasant situations. Professionals are attracted to the healthcare industry usually because they want to care for others and be respected for their contribution. The shift from people to profits has seriously contaminated the characteristics of the workplace that control followership; confusion among priorities seems to be driving much of today's difficulty. When we enter a particular setting, certain stimuli prompt or cue our behavior. If we walk into a church, for example, we become quiet, but if we walk into a football stadium, we are able to yell and cheer. It is the environmental context, then, that makes behavior appropriate or inappropriate. If someone behaved in church as if he or she were in a stadium, that person would be considered inappropriate at the very least and possibly crazy.

Healthcare executives face a similar situation. They must discover how to create a clear context that allows followers to behave in ways that reinforce the reasons they originally entered the profession. Most men and women choose healthcare as a profession because they feel confident and secure that, no matter what their function, they will work in a context of caring and compassion. Patients enter the delivery system expecting the same. However, the emphasis on money during the last 20-plus years changed the rules of conduct and transformed the context for working in healthcare. Executives who once worked in the altruistic context of service to the community now must concern themselves with market share, physician competition, downsizing, consolidation, and diversification. The effect on potential followers is that they hear the message, "Of course you can care and heal, just do it within the budget." Imagine how this message is perceived among staff. Am I nothing more than an economic unit? At what point does my performance cost more than it is worth? Executives, physicians, nurses, other caregivers, and support staff began to question their role in healthcare. Furthermore, they began to wonder why they chose a career in healthcare as attitudes, beliefs, roles, and leadership and management styles seemed to come under constant attack. Is there any question why medical school and nursing school enrollment continues to decline?

Potential followers exhibit some common reactions to the multitude of pressures in today's healthcare work environment.

- *Regression.* Insecure and afraid because of the seemingly constant changes in expectations, staff cling to tradition and revert to nostalgic discussions about "the good old days."

- *Aggression.* Angry and frustrated by the change in context, staff lash out at everything that represents the new order. They (especially the physicians) may openly refuse to cooperate and may even resort to sabotage.
- *Passivity.* Confused by the mixed messages so common in today's workplace, staff may tolerate new initiatives but remain skeptical, suspicious, and detached from the change process.
- *Apathy.* An extension of passivity is apathy—the total lack of caring. Constant frustration breeds anger, and continued frustration beyond anger results in apathy. This complete lack of commitment is the most difficult condition in which to engage followers.
- *Symbolism.* Baffled by the changes in the context for working in healthcare, staff develop an almost neurotic obsession with making symbolic gestures. They confuse activity with outcome. For example, committees and task forces are created to identify or study the problems. Meeting rituals are seen as being responsive but deliver no measurable improvements.
- *Grouping.* Alienated and isolated by the changes in context, staff turn to others for support, encouragement, and protection. "It's us against them," peers assure each other. Clearly, this behavior is reflected in increased union activity and strong antiadministration reactions from physicians.
- *Leadership.* Challenged by the change in context, the rare individuals who respond as leaders give the new economic context meaning and craft clear messages that are understandable to the workforce. "This is the situation, and this is what it means for us," they tell their followers. "Here are some ideas about how we can work together to turn these challenges into an opportunity to create an even more effective organization."

Greg Carlson is a leader who exemplifies the last bullet point above. As president and CEO of Owensboro Mercy Health System in Kentucky since this merged entity was created in 1994, he has anchored his leadership in the following six "core commitments" or corporate values: integrity, service, respect, teamwork, excellence, and innovation. Carlson bases his decision making on the consideration of one or more of these values, and his faithfulness to them has created a powerful corporate culture in which followers flourish (see Chapter 8 for change process description and data). Herein lies the most significant difference between executives in title only (those who are unable to inspire followers) and leaders (those who have followers). The titled healthcare executives will only respond to a change in context by acquiring tools, programs, and gadgets to fix the problems caused by the change. They will read books on high-performance organizations and rigidly practice "executive rituals" to project an illusion of dynamism and credibility. Caught in the grip of their own illusions, they assume that if they act, dress, and talk like real leaders, staff will follow them. Substance is replaced by form.

True leaders dress themselves in the corporate values. The physical and verbal behavior of Carlson and other effective healthcare leaders can be related directly to one or more of the six core values he espouses. It is the consistency of values-based behaviors that inspires followers.

Behavioral consistency places all change in a clear context of values. Patrick Lencioni (2000, 152), as mentioned in his book *The Four Obsessions of an Extraordinary Executive,** believes successful executives obsess about "organizational clarity." He states, "An

> "With increasing workforce and reimbursement challenges in an environment of physician demands for either significant equity or participation in the core programs or revenues that generate hospital profits, LEADERSHIP will be challenged at all levels of the organization from the board room to the CEO to all management . . . the surviving and thriving healthcare organizations will have aligned and stable leadership—with values consistently applied and demonstrated throughout the organization."
>
> —*Hans Wiik, FACHE, president and CEO, Health Future, LLC, Ashland, Oregon*

---

* Material from *The Four Obsessions of an Extraordinary Executive* by Patrick Lencioni. Copyright © 2000, John Wiley & Sons. This material is used by permission of John Wiley & Sons, Inc.

organization that has achieved clarity has a sense of unity around everything it does. It aligns its resources, especially the human ones, around common concepts, values, definitions, goals, and strategies, thereby realizing the synergies that all great companies must achieve. The result is an undeniable sense of focus and efficiency, concepts even the most quantitatively oriented leader can embrace. Employees in these organizations seem to have amazing levels of autonomy." The employees at Owensboro Mercy Health System have a great deal of freedom, but it is a freedom within a clear set of values-based behaviors. One of Carlson's most frequent quotes, which he related to me in an interview, is, "Leaders create expectations, they inspire, they create a vision, they model the values, and, most importantly, they trust others to make decisions within the context of the vision and values. True leaders are willing to take chances, make mistakes, and create an environment where people have fun."

Donald N. Sull (2000) depicts ineffective leaders in an excellent article entitled "Why Good Companies Go Bad." In this article, Sull coins the phrase *active intertia* to explain why some titled executives increasingly behave in ways that have no effect or a negative effect on what they claim to be the goal: "The fresh thinking that led to a company's initial success is replaced by a rigid devotion to the status quo. And when changes occur in the company's markets, the formula that had brought success instead brings failure" (Sull 2000, 5). The belief is that what worked in the past is still valid—it just needs to be executed more often and faster. This is active inertia, where more is done but no movement takes place.

This belief is in stark contrast to the behavior of those who focus on followership. Followers want a consistent message; they want to know how to move from the past to the present and know their specific role in building the bridge to the future. Followers will embrace the anxiety, frustration, and uncertainty of the tasks because the person they follow can turn fear of change into confidence about the future.

Healthcare professionals universally acknowledge that this industry is no longer a comfortable or predictable field, but unfortunately, several titled executives still are unaware that growing followership is the solution to their difficulties. Most remain blinded by the quantitative, tangible issues that flood their desk. They tend to focus on the content of the immediate crisis, not on a context of behavior and decision making about the future. One crisis after another arises, and the titled executives obsess about them instead of addressing and preventing them. Challenged by constant change and escalating demands, they become tyrannized by day-to-day problems. Like the sirens in *Ulysses,* problems come to have a mysterious and seductive power over titled executives who, like the sailors in that epic story, can easily end up on the rocks, dazed and bewildered by their loss of control.

> "Leaders must look down the road, always setting direction by communicating their vision to the organization. This has become my way of life. There is not any encounter with staff that we don't leave without asking if our actions help us pursue the vision. We then communicate each action showing how it leads to achieving success and meeting the vision."
>
> —*Kelly Mather, CEO, Sutter Lakeside Hospital, Lakeport, California*

When titled executives become seduced by immediate, tangible, quantitative problems, they respond with one or more of the predictable response patterns discussed in the following sections.

The Detail Trap

For some people, data and details assume the power of a cult ritual. The behavior of titled executives caught in this trap is dominated by such statements as, "We need more data" or "We are still analyzing the data, and until we understand it more completely, we can't move ahead." These executives do not have followers because they are unresponsive to the needs of the employees—because they need more data on the correct way to respond! The executive believes the myth that obsessing over the details of data is a mark of the serious and tough-minded executive. In reality, the resulting "analysis paralysis" cripples progress. It permits the executive to live in a safe, no-lose world where blame for any problem rests with those who pushed for a decision too quickly, before the data were analyzed completely.

In "Quotations from Powell: A Leadership Primer," the appendix to Oren Harari's (2002) book *The Leadership Secrets of Colin Powell,* Secretary of State Powell provides 18 lessons in leadership. Lesson 15 advises how to avoid the detail trap, stating, "Part I: Use the formula P = 40 to 70, in which P stands for the probability of success and the numbers indicate the percentage of information acquired. Part II: Once the information is in the 40 to 70 range, go with your gut."

The Totality Trap

Another group of titled executives operates at the opposite extreme. Seduced by the magic of cosmic macrothinking, they tell the potential followers, "I'm studying the issue. I can't decide until I understand the totality of the impact." As with the detail trap, this approach leads to paralysis, in this case because the future can never be defined enough for a commitment to be made. For that very reason, the titled executive is allowed to avoid making a decision because the solutions depend on a perfect understanding of an unknowable future. Without the courage to commit, these executives will produce no followers.

The Micro/Macro Trap

Not content with a single world view, titled executives alternate between seeing their environment as atomic particles and as the

Milky Way. On Monday, this type of executive might say to the director of planning and marketing, "This is a great idea, but give me the details. I need to see the numbers." Eager to move forward toward a final decision, the director returns with the numbers by Friday only to hear, "OK, now can you help me see the big picture? I want to know where this is going in the next five years." These executives never feel pressured to make a decision because whatever position is proposed, they can take a counter position.

Consider the effects of this approach on the subordinates and other employees of executives caught in this trap. Rather than asking what is best for the organization, they are more apt to think, I'd better be ready to defend myself. Ultimately, subordinates grow weary of being whipsawed by this retrogressive game and quit innovating. They also do not become followers of this kind of executive. More likely they ridicule the inability of the boss to focus and decide. Why do titled healthcare executives run their staff through mazes of contradictory conditions? Perhaps they feel impotent in the face of issues, such as quality, regulation, financial risk, competition, and all of the other components defining today's healthcare industry, which is characterized by accelerating and unpredictable change. Reeling from changes in regulation and reimbursement that never seem to abate, they choose a course of overcontrolling people, information, and final decision making. With this strategy, they control their subordinates with minutiae (microthinking) and lock their boards into a permanent holding pattern with macrothinking.

Sooner or later the board chairperson, the president of the medical staff, or perhaps a competitor will unveil the truth that the head of the organization is incapable of making a courageous decision. In the wake of this realization, staff do not follow titled executives. They live in the delusion that they were leading, but no one was following.

The Checklist Trap

Titled executives seem to be powerfully inclined to invest time and energy in tasks for which they have a good track record. If their financial reports have received rave reviews from the board, they will continue to churn them out. This repetition of successful and highly praised behaviors is, of course, human nature. However, potential followers will easily determine that the priority of the titled executive is self-preservation, not courageous leadership. These executives operate on the assumption that personal success is a byproduct of the number of "things to do." The more cluttered the calendar, the more pressing the deadlines, the more important they feel. What if these titled executives could rid themselves of their to-do lists? Would they really take advantage of that freed-up time to inspire followers? Not likely. Given their perception of self-importance, they would probably invent new and different, but still meaningless, things to do.

> "It is critical that leaders 'look down the road.' Too often our decisions are focused on the present due to pressures from boards, physicians, and community. Not all health-care leaders are frightened by the future. Those who can shape their future feel more secure than those who let things happen."
>
> —*Richard C. Breon*, FACHE, *president and* CEO, *Spectrum Health, Grand Rapids, Michigan*

Titled executives perform tasks and execute procedures. Leaders spend time creating a corporate culture with such clarity and focus that their followers not only understand how to act but why they should act in those certain ways. Leaders give work meaning—a context. It is this dynamic that inspires others to follow them.

Take a look at your calendar for the previous week and answer the following questions:

1. How much time did you spend solving problems or resolving crises?

2. How much time did you spend addressing financial issues?
3. Compare the time you invested in solving problems and discussing finance with the time you spent on developing followers. How much time did you spend communicating the mission and vision? How much time did you spend re-recruiting those staff who most exemplify the corporate values? How much time did you spend measuring and managing the intangibles that underpin organizational excellence?

Another easy leadership audit is to analyze phone usage.

1. Who do you call most often? Why?
2. Who do you avoid or postpone calling? What calls do you delegate to others?
3. How much time do you spend on which calls? Why?

Based on your analysis of both your calendar and your phone calls, what conclusions can you reach about your investment in human capital versus financial capital? How do you cope with problems involving the organization's mission, values, and vision? To what extent are you a victim of the traps of detail, totality, and micro/macro thinking? Have followers increased their commitment because of how you used your time, talent, and energy?

We are our behavior. Personal investment is measured by where time is spent. Healthcare executives who are leaders—that is, who have the most followers—are those with the most personal investment in human capital.

KNOW WHERE YOU ARE GOING AND WHO IS GOING WITH YOU

Healthcare executives with a large number of followers understand two fundamental concepts:

1. Staff will follow those who are able to communicate an inspirational vision.
2. Leaders are successful to the degree that they surround themselves with the right people.

Jim Collins and Jerry Porras's (1994) book *Built to Last: Successful Habits of Visionary Companies* makes a strong case about those organizations that are successful over a long period of time (perhaps 50 years or more). They posit that this degree of success is a function of the correct vision and how the vision is communicated. In a more recent text, *Good to Great: Why Some Companies Make the Leap . . . and Others Don't,* Jim Collins (2001, 13)† modifies this notion with the idea that the critical success element in sustainable success is less the vision and more the people.

> First Who . . . Then What. We expected that the good-to-great leaders would begin by setting a new vision and strategy. We found instead that they first got the right people on the bus, the wrong people off the bus, and the right people in the right seats—and then they figured out where to drive it. The old adage, "People are your most important asset," turns out to be wrong. People are not your most important asset. The right people are.

The role of the symphony conductor is a good analogy for that of a healthcare leader who is able to inspire followers. First, the conductor selects the best players for each instrument and chair. Then he or she selects the score. If the score (or the health system) needs to change (e.g., because of a market, regulatory, or reimbursement change), these highly skilled performers are able to adjust. Leaders know why they are there: to inspire. They select

---

† Material from *Good to Great: Why Some Companies Make the Leap . . . and Others Don't* by Jim Collins. Copyright © 2001 by Jim Collins. Reprinted with permission from Jim Collins and HarperCollins Publishers Inc.

and communicate the score, always making sure, of course, that their musicians are skilled enough to handle the music and any adaptations to it. Leaders know that they cannot use their precious time solving problems as they arise. They let the managers worry about the present and the immediate past; leaders must always look ahead, always set and fine tune the direction, with complete trust in the skills and motivation of those around them.

Healthcare leaders today need to select the right team, see the future, communicate clear expectations, and live the values. This simple formula for success is extremely difficult to consistently apply in our highly competitive and regulated environment. Leaders are confronted with a daily dose of what can be characterized as cataclysmic changes. Revenue margins will continue to shrink, capital will be harder to acquire, the problems associated with physician relations will continue, and the vacancies of healthcare professions caused by the current shortages will need to be filled. These are some of the key pressure points confronting today's leaders. The amount of discipline and courage required to transcend these dynamics is immense.

Many suffer from the corrosive effects of these factors if they are not treated successfully. Some titled executives lose their jobs, move into early retirement, or begin second careers. Even those who are currently at the helm of healthcare organizations seldom feel confident and secure. Instead, they candidly, but privately, describe themselves as threatened, angry, and confused about their profession and their career.

Yet there is a group of healthcare leaders who thrive in this seemingly chaotic environment. What differentiates these two groups is a transcendent purpose that allows their staff the opportunity to subordinate their self-interests for a greater good. The staffs of those leaders who construct and communicate this transcendent purpose become followers. This is the gift and the genius of leaders. They present a picture of a world that is better than the one that exists currently. They address the realities of the sacrifices needed to create this world. They explain the role of the followers. They ignite the process of reaching the transcendent purpose with hope.

In the broadest sense, as defined by Donald Graber and James Johnson (2001, 40), there is a spiritual aspect to the process of creating followers. "A common theme is that one's search for spiritual growth and fulfillment need not be separate from one's work. Spirituality implies an inner search for meaning or fulfillment that may be taken by any one, regardless of religion." All of the world's great leaders were able to convince large numbers of people that their long-term self-interests would be best served by subordinating their current needs for a greater good. Christ, Gandhi, Napoleon, Abraham Lincoln, Martin Luther King, Jr., and Mother Teresa all created followers who believed that these individuals would make their life better.

> "It is not who you know or even what you know. It is who has the fortitude to implement good, hard-to-make decisions with humanity and sensitivity."
>
> —*Wayne Lerner, DR.P.H., FACHE, president and CEO, Rehabilitation Institute of Chicago*

Followers flourish in a workplace that balances the tangible and the intangible factors of that environment. Staff will follow someone who achieves predictable results and respects the efforts of those who did the work. Leaders understand that they will have followers as long as they produce results and show respect. Figure 1.1 shows the main elements of the tangibles and the intangibles and includes in that paradigm the increasingly important "corporate soul." The three domains of tangibles, intangibles, and the corporate soul must always be in balance in work environments that promote followership. The use of the corporate soul in the grid shown in Figure 1.1 is a modification of its description in Eric Klein and John Izzo's (1999) book *Awakening Corporate Soul*. In this grid, the corporate soul is defined as the boundary between the tangibles and the intangibles. The need to measure and manage each of the inputs and outputs is well understood by leaders. Titled executives tend to focus only on the tangibles.

The elements in Figure 1.1 are separated into inputs and outputs. Since the mid-1980s, titled executives have become very adroit at measuring and managing the tangibles. Too often this obsession with short-term tangible increases has been at the expense of the intangibles and the corporate soul.

The tangible elements are very familiar and therefore need no definitions. However, the intangibles and corporate soul elements are many times misunderstood. The role of the leader in this domain is to provide meaning to work; show that all staff, patients, and other community members are cared for; and give to the staff those things that make their work effective.

When leaders provide meaning, caring, and giving, followers emerge because they feel a sense of purpose, joy, and pride in the profession and with their employer. The techniques that leaders use to provide meaning, caring, and giving vary widely. Several of the more successful techniques are described later in this book.

The intangible inputs and outputs can be the cause of many profound discussions among titled executives. These discussions typically are stimulated by a critical mass of negative data about the outputs. Titled executives are especially sensitive to negative data about morale, job satisfaction, trust, and so forth because they seem to believe that the intangibles should take care of themselves and that time must be spent instead on the tangibles (e.g., finance). Leaders, on the other hand, know that their main job is to sustain the inspiration of followers. This is only possible by rigorous measurement and management of the intangibles.

Leaders are also aware that it is the strength of the intangibles that drives the success in the tangibles. Two non-healthcare examples are Wal-Mart and Southwest Airlines. Why is Wal-Mart the number one Fortune 500 company on the basis of sales and K-Mart filed bankruptcy? Why has Southwest Airlines continued to be profitable year after year and United Airlines filed bankruptcy? Sam Walton, founder of Wal-Mart, and Herb Kelleher, cofounder of Southwest Airlines, knew that the tangibles and the

Figure 1.1: The Three Work Environment Domains

	TANGIBLES	*CORPORATE SOUL*	*INTANGIBLES*
INPUTS	• Cash	• Meaning	• Mission
	• People	• Caring	• Values
	• Policy/Procedures	• Giving	• Vision
	• Strategy		• Inspiration
	• Plant		• Leadership Style
	• Information		• Recognition
	• Systems		• Motivation
	• Communications		
OUTPUTS	• Profit	• Inner Peace of Purpose	• Culture
	• Market Share	• Joy	• Commitment
	• Customer	• Pride	• Followers
	• Satisfaction		• Job
	• Growth		• Satisfaction
	• Productivity		• Team Spirit
	• Quality		• Trust
			• Quality

Source: Atchison, T. 2001. "Striking a Balance." *Trustee* 54 (7): 28. Reprinted from *Trustee*, Vol. 54 No. 7, by permission, July/August 2001, Copyright 2001, by Health Forum, Inc.

intangibles must be balanced. True leaders know the true mantra for success: no balance, no business.

CONCLUSION

What the healthcare industry is now experiencing is nothing short of the collapse of the old order. Many of the rules for success that have worked for so many years no longer work. Today's healthcare leaders must master a new set of behaviors that balances the tangibles and the intangibles if they are to create a work environment that in turn creates followers. Leaders inspire followers to unleash their potential for the greater good of providing quality care to the community.

REFERENCES

Atchison, T. "Striking a Balance." *Trustee* 54 (7): 28.

Carlson, G. 2002. Interview with author.

Collins, J. 2001. *Good to Great: Why Some Companies Make the Leaps . . . and Others Don't*. New York: HarperCollins.

Collins, J., and J. Porras. 1994. *Built to Last: Successful Habits of Visionary Companies*. New York: HarperCollins.

Graber, D. R., and J. A. Johnson. 2001. "Spirituality and Healthcare Organizations." *Journal of Healthcare Management* 46 (1): 39–50.

Harari, O. 2002. *The Leadership Secrets of Colin Powell*. New York: McGraw-Hill.

Klein, E., and J. B. Izzo. 1999. *Awakening Corporate Soul: Four Paths to Unleash the Power of People at Work*. Gloucester, MA: Fair Winds Press.

Lencioni, P. 2000. *The Four Obsessions of an Extraordinary Executive*. San Francisco: Jossey-Bass.

Sull, D. N. 2000. "Why Good Companies Go Bad." *Harvard Business Review* 77 (4): 42–48, 50–52, 183.

CHAPTER 2

Bridging Myth and Reality

FOLLOWERS THRIVE IN very specific ecosystems. Leaders understand that the best way to produce followers is to create a work environment that aligns personal values and skills with corporate values and work requirements. James L. Reinertsen, M.D., head of The Reinertsen Group, a consulting firm that helps healthcare leaders create organizational environments in which health professionals can grow and flourish, is quoted as saying, "If you want to create a rhinoceros, you must simultaneously create the treed Savannah" (Reinertsen 1999). In other words, nurturing environments precede the creation of life forms.

Some leadership literature, such as *Fish! A Remarkable Way to Boost Morale and Improve Results* (Lundin, Paul, and Christensen 2000), provide suggestions on where to start building followership. However, little has been written on how to manage the deeper process of building a corporate culture based on the core values and measurable workplace goals that sustains a "fun, energizing" place to work such as the kind that *Fish!* promotes. The process of identifying the level of followership an organization currently experiences and creating a follower-friendly work environment is found in the measurement and management of corporate cultures. (For the purposes of this book, a strong corporate culture is defined as the environment created by leaders that results in nurturing followers.)

Creating a strong corporate culture takes a big commitment from the trustees and the senior executives of the organization. The consistently high level of commitment required to establish a healthy work environment is very difficult in today's complicated healthcare industry. Because we are creatures of habit, we tend to be uneasy about the unpredictability of change—especially a big change like transforming a corporate culture. We tend to find reasons not to change. In doing so, we avoid any data that support change and enthusiastically embrace any data that support the status quo. Many of the reasons to resist change are embedded in some widely held myths about corporate culture.

Myths of Mission

"We need a mission that protects our not-for-profit status, so let the lawyers write it." Protecting a not-for-profit status is a noble goal, but it may have little or nothing to do with the organization's mission—that is, with its reason for existence. A self-protective statement drafted by attorneys will do nothing to enhance commitment, motivate staff, or help employees focus on vision.

"Mission statements are for the community, not for management." A mission statement answers one important question: Why does this organization exist? Unless healthcare executives know and understand their purpose, they will find themselves trapped in defensive positions. While a mission statement may have meaning to external audiences, it is not really written for the community. For example, community leaders may read the mission statement and change their image of the organization, but in con-

trast to physicians, trustees, employees, and managers, community residents will never live the mission in their daily lives.

"Mission statements should be lofty, eloquent, and long." A mission statement should not contain more than three or four basic ideas, and these ideas should be easy to remember. They should be expressed skillfully but in "plain speak" and in short, tight sentences. The best mission statements distill the essence of the organization.

"Mission statements must be idealistic." If a mission statement is idealistic, it becomes ineffective. Instead, the mission statement should define in very specific terms why the organization exists. If the statement incorporates such value-laden words as *charity* and *healing,* the workforce must see a close connection between the language of the statement and what they do on the job. They must understand how they make the organization's mission come alive.

"Mission statements are worthless. They have little practical value in day-to-day management." If a mission statement is idealistic and impractical, it is indeed worthless. However, when a mission statement focuses on an organization's real reason for existence, it becomes the acid text for all decisions, including hiring, allocating capital, formulating the budget, expanding or reducing service lines, downsizing, strategic planning, and, most importantly, developing board policy.

H. Lee Moffitt Cancer Center in Tampa, Florida, is an exceptional example of how a mission statement underpins all decisions and as a result sets the stage for a very follower-friendly environment in a high-performing organization. Moffitt's mission is "To contribute to the prevention and cure of cancer." This mission statement is short, easy to remember, and very meaningful to the trustees, executives, managers, other employees, physicians, scientists, and volunteers. When concerns about fiscal matters, human resources challenges, or market shifts arise, these nine words provide the context for decision making. All other considerations are irrelevant. Moffitt's mission statement charges the organization to do nothing more than help patients afflicted with cancer and ultimately find cures.

"Why bother with a mission statement? Employees never understand them anyway." It is true that in the past mission statements were often misunderstood by everyone in the organization, including executives and trustees. But when leaders properly communicate the mission, every follower in the organization—from the board chairperson to the nurse's aide—will understand the statement and be able to apply it to job performance.

> "Real leadership has nothing to do with titles or position. The job of the leader is to live the mission and values as well as communicate the vision in ways that the expectations are clear—and then, get out of the way and let others lead."
>
> —*Greg Carlson,* CHE, *president and* CEO, *Owensboro Mercy Health System, Owensboro, Kentucky*

"Trustees cannot function without traditional mission statements." Trustees generally preferred long and lofty mission statements that celebrated the organization's traditions and history—and some still maintain that bias. As a result, many organizations now supplement their mission statements with statements that set forth their philosophy, standards, or principles. These statements should echo the organization's core values.

The ideal mission statement, however, should be clear and direct, as, for example, "We exist to provide a continuum of high-quality care to the residents of our community." In addition, the mission statement should be used as the first criterion or standard for making decisions. If an organization exists to provide a continuum of high-quality care to community residents, it would resist investments in regional medical care programs and instead might pursue opportunities in home care, long-term care, or women's health.

Many mission statements incorporate the organization's core values. These values are the convictions that drive all behavior, and it is only when the core corporate values and the fundamental personal values of the employees come together that strong followership emerges. Without solid grounding in a values-based mission, employees may fulfill job requirements, but they will do little to make the organization more effective. When staff members function outside the context of the values-based mission, they may or may not support the organization. Their primary goal may be simply to do their job and get a paycheck.

Myths of Motivation

Myths of motivation, the why and how people work and function, are grounded in misperceptions of followership. In confronting and exploding the following myths, healthcare leaders should look within themselves to ascertain what personal traits, experiences, or attitudes are allowing them to rely on these myths as crutches and thereby reducing the number of followers.

"Most employees are motivated by money." In reality, most employees are motivated by personal feelings of self-worth. In some organizations, however, the only way employees feel any self-worth is through their paychecks. But money as a motivator has several limitations. Money functions as an incentive on only one level, and it is a disincentive on two others. Money is an incentive when it fits employees' perception of their worth. However, if compensation is perceived as too low, employees will feel used. At the same time, if compensation is far beyond the employee's skills and the position's perceived market value, employees will fear that they may lose their job if they are ever "discovered." In addition, their sense of self-esteem will inevitably erode if they feel they are not earning what they are being paid.

In general, the motivational effect of financial compensation is inversely related to the amount of respect that employees receive. The more employees are mistreated or ignored, the more they demand higher pay. This relationship between respect and money is one of the most misunderstood causes of motivational ineffectiveness in healthcare organizations.

"Some people cannot be motivated." The reality is that everyone is 100 percent motivated 100 percent of the time. Everyone has a full reservoir of motivation. The caveat is that people may not be motivated to do what the organization wants them to do. A nurse, for example, may, for reasons not necessarily related to the organization's expectations, be highly motivated to organize his or her unit, socialize with other nurses, or pick arguments with physicians. A dietitian may be motivated to do very little because of negative incentives: "If I try something new, I'll get yelled at, but if I maintain the status quo, my manager will leave me alone." In the same way, an admitting clerk will glance at his or her paycheck and conclude, "If I work really hard, I will get a 3 percent raise. But if I continue working at the same pace, I will probably still get a 3 percent raise." The lesson is clear: If tangible and intangible rewards and recognition are scarce, employees typically see no reason to alter or enhance their behavior. Unfortunately, the titled executive may conclude that staff members are simply not motivated to do new things; they are not risk takers. In reality, the employees may be risk takers who are trapped in an organization that offers no reasons for taking risks but does offer significant reasons for avoiding them.

If employees are motivated to organize collective bargaining units, they will use their time, talent, and energy to force management to do their bidding. They could instead use their time, talent, and energy to fulfill the organization's mission, support its values, and achieve its vision. To produce the latter result, titled executives must become leaders and create an environment in which organizing a bargaining unit becomes unthinkable for employees. The real issue, then, is not how to motivate but how to *direct* and *manage* the motivation of managers, trustees, physicians, and employees.

"Motivation never lasts." In fact, behaviors do burn out and enthusiasm wanes when employees are driven exclusively by external rewards. However, followers sustain performance because they internalize behavior and accept it as their own. Indeed, once

followers have internalized a behavior, they will maintain it under the most difficult circumstances. By contrast, if external factors such as money or fear are used exclusively to provide motivation, performance will ebb and flow in direct relationship to the presence or absence of the reward or threat. For example, a primary care nurse who works in the emergency room simply because she is paid a premium will probably never perform at the same level as a nurse who believes that the emergency room is the most exciting area of the hospital.

"People need to be continually motivated." Again, all people are motivated 100 percent of the time. Motivation cannot be created; it can only be directed. The best way to direct motivation is to match the values and goals of the organization to the individual's values. When followers see "the good" in their work, they perform at high levels because the result is greater benefits to all. They feel they are a part of something bigger than themselves.

"Staff motivation takes too much time." Unleashing and directing motivation may indeed take a great deal of time and money if the goal is to perform the organizational equivalent of shifting the axis of the earth. For example, if the goal is to help the medical director behave more like an executive, it may take a long time to achieve that goal. Whether it is worth the time depends on how much that physician will help fulfill the organization's mission. However, working with key leaders to improve one small staff behavior a month is easy. Leaders think small, move fast, and celebrate often. When starting a new service, leaders set small, achievable goals so followership grows as people gain confidence in their new responsibilities. Even daily goals may be prudent in the beginning.

"In the present healthcare environment, it takes longer to motivate employees." Despite pressures from business, government, payers, and consumers, motivation takes no more time today than it did in the years before prospective payment. In today's environment, motivating people to adapt to change just seems to take longer because the pace and volume of change is increased. Titled

executives are frightened and rush to reestablish control to give themselves a sense (illusion) of security. If they do this in the midst of chaos, their employees will seek safety by circling their wagons and digging their trenches, effectively shutting out senior management.

"The only real motives are fear and greed." In reality, the only things that direct motivation over time are consistency of values and role clarity. A strong culture has many followers because it offers clearly understood roles, a bridge between past and present expectations, and support for taking risks and moving ahead to achieve the organization's vision. In a weak culture, however, employees are often confused about what management expects and wants, and they fail to understand why the old way is no longer adequate. Fearing reprimand, they avoid innovation and risk taking, perpetuating the weak culture. Fear and greed are the tools of the weak and only create a toxic work environment. On the other hand, matching what employees value with what the organization values is a way of directing motivation and creating a nurturing environment.

"Employees can't be treated the same way as managers." In reality, the more employees understand the organization's mission, accept its values, and share in the achievement of its vision, the deeper will be their commitment to the organization. If employees feel disenfranchised, they will stay around for their paychecks and may even modify their behavior if threatened with termination. But the data processing manager, the accountant, and the quality assurance coordinator will perform at top levels only when they understand how they make a difference to the organization. It must be impressed on the parking garage attendant that friendly greetings to patrons are important to the hospital's reputation for high-quality service, and the person who delivers food trays to patients must understand how hot or cold food can affect the overall perception of care.

"With some people, motivation is the carrot; with others, it is the stick." People can be motivated temporarily to carry out difficult

or unattractive activities through a balance of rewards and threats. In an effective healthcare organization, however, carrots and sticks both become unnecessary because people understand how they fit into the organization and contribute to its goals. Healthcare leaders must give meaningful recognition to the achievements of employees and minimize the threat of punishment. Self-managed employees create their own "internal" carrots and sticks.

Myths of Titled Executives

Myths of mission and motivation shape and direct myths of management such as those that follow. If titled executives believe that a mission statement is little more than window dressing and that people are little more than interchangeable parts of a (not necessarily) well-oiled machine, they will cling to the outmoded concepts of titled executive behavior. They will view their role as managing material assets rather than human assets, and, while they may build bigger organizations, they will not make them more effective.

> "I remember when we used to think that our mission statement had to be long, lofty, and somehow poetic. That was a silly idea, because it was too hard to keep people focused upon what was really important . . . they were too busy trying to remember the prose."
>
> —Robert Bonar, PH.D., president and CEO, Children's Hospital of Austin, Texas

Healthcare leaders have one purpose: To increase followers by building commitment to the organization's mission, values, and vision. But this requires that followers understand who they are, the purpose of their work, and how they can contribute to the success of the organization. Followers crave the intangible locus of control found in a values-based mission as well as a vision they can accept and apply to their work lives. In this, the role of healthcare leadership is critical. If those in charge treat staff like machines and continually look for new buttons to push, staff will behave like machines and perform—but only until they fulfill the minimum requirements of an assignment. If they have both responsibility and freedom, they will perform for the organization, not just for themselves.

"Top management does not have time to worry about people." The reality is that just as a symphony conductor worries about the score and having the right musicians, leaders invest their time creating an environment that will heighten the contribution of the followers. When titled executives are continually obsessed with buildings, financial reports, and legal briefs, employees quickly get the message that "what we do here does not really make a difference." The response from employees is, "If executives want to worry only about money and projects, we'll organize a union. If management won't talk to us as individuals, they will have to talk to us as a bargaining unit." Titled executives who have no time to worry about people may be forced to take time when a collective bargaining unit is recognized or when people leave in large numbers. When employees feel exploited, they will not commit to the organization. When they feel some ownership, however, anything that does not help the organization seems like a waste of time.

"My role is to build an organization." The reality is that an organization's greatest asset is not its strategic plan or balance sheet but its human capital. Thomas J. Watson (1963, 5–6) made the following statement while serving as president of IBM:*

> I firmly believe that any organization, in order to survive and achieve success, must have a sound set of beliefs on which it premises all of its policies and actions.
>
> Next I believe that the most important single factor in corporate success is faithful adherence to those beliefs.
>
> And finally, I believe that if an organization is to meet the challenge of a changing world, it must be prepared to change

---

* Thomas J. Watson, *A Business and Its Beliefs: The Ideas that Helped Build IBM,* copyright © 1963, McGraw-Hill. This material is reproduced with permission of The McGraw-Hill Companies.

everything about itself except those beliefs as it moves through corporate life.

In other words, the basic philosophy, spirit, and drive of an organization have far more to do with its relative achievements than do technological or economic resources, organizational structure, innovation, and timing. All these weigh heavily in success. But they are, I think, transcended by how strongly the people in the organization believe in its precepts and how faithfully they carry them out.

"Loyalty cannot be created." Leaders generate loyalty by being consistent. If you show care and concern for people, they will respond in the same way. Recently, a healthcare system closed down a hospital, moved employees 20 miles away to another hospital, and still increased commitment and job satisfaction in the workforce. How? On day one, the CEO stood before his employees and said, "No one will get hurt. No one will lose his or her pension, and to the best of our ability, no one will leave here professionally damaged. However, we need to shut down this hospital and move most of you to a new hospital across town. Some of you won't go. Some of you may not want to go. We want to do this as fairly and compassionately as possible. So let's work together."

Following this meeting, the organization turned to its values-based mission to help employees understand the importance of closing the hospital. As a result, each follower could conclude that "the community is better for me losing my job in this location; a good greater than my interests is being served."

LEADING OTHERS BY MANAGING CHANGE

The leader's primary role is to build a strong culture by modeling the organization's mission, values, and vision. This sets the tone for interaction within the workforce. The goal is to create an organization of self-managed people who understand their role in fulfilling the organization's values-based mission and achieving its vision. The effective healthcare leader communicates the purpose of the organization to each one of the followers—from the chairperson of the board to the security guard to the physical therapist.

Consider an example. Does a mother, a father, two children, a house in the suburbs, and two cars add up to a family? Not necessarily, unless the members of the family are united by bonds of love and trust. Something similar is true of healthcare organizations. The mere fact that a hospital has a CEO, a board, a medical staff, and strategic and financial plans does not make it an effective hospital. Like strong and happy families, effective organizations have shared values, a "magical" quality, a spirit—a strong culture based on shared beliefs and common goals. Ideas emerge and the organization moves forward because of the underlying values that pervade and sustain everyone involved.

It is often said that the best teams are not necessarily those with the best athletes but those with the best coaches. Like the winning coach, the healthcare leader is pivotal in creating and building meaning for the workforce. Again and again, the following scenario takes place: A leader leaves an organization, and another competent professional takes her place. No one knows why, but things are never quite the same again. "I don't know what's going on," moans the new hospital vice president. "I'm doing everything my predecessor did, but I'm not getting the same results." What this executive failed to realize is that the first leader gave the organization something intangible: inspiration, *esprit de corps,* camaraderie, and a sense of pride and joy that can never be replicated by simply adhering to policies and procedures.

For many healthcare executives, focusing their organization on issues such as mission, values, and vision will not be easy. If you find that to be true of yourself, try to keep the following concepts in mind.

Change is a process, not an event. It involves much more than creating a new business venture or delegating a pet project. When it comes to changing management styles, quick fixes never work.

Such changes are far more complicated than installing a new software package or telephone system. Instead, you are trying to change people, many of whom have practiced the same behaviors for decades.

Change is a personal experience. Not everyone in the organization will respond to it in the same way. Nurses may embrace your efforts, while those in finance may ridicule it as "soft stuff." Be prepared to adapt your change program to the followers' needs and idiosyncrasies.

Change is experiential. The reality of change cannot be communicated through memos, slide presentations, videos, or brochures. Change will occur only when people experience the process and sense the excitement that comes from reshaping an organization. The more meaningful experiences people share, the more they will change their feelings and behaviors.

Change must be expressed in practical, how-to terms. The key to successful change is helping members of the workforce understand what change can mean for them. In what new ways will they perform their jobs? Will they feel differently about their coworkers? What problems will they attempt to solve? Leaders always clarify roles and expectations.

Keep the process simple. No matter how many workbooks are purchased, no matter how many seminars or lectures are sponsored, the final responsibility for change rests with the individual.

> "In almost 30 years of working with and for people, my biggest disappointment was in a CEO I liked and admired who voiced one standard and personally violated that standard. Leaders must inspire 100 percent of the time through their words and behaviors."
>
> —Ron Ommen, FACHE, CEO, St. John's Medical Center, Jackson, Wyoming

In the midst of the change process, it is not uncommon for titled healthcare executives to regress to past management styles. To offset that inclination, create a team of "organizational spotters"—that is, trusted colleagues who understand the necessity of changing the organization. If your leadership style does begin to regress, these spotters can provide confidential feedback on how, when, and where the change process fell off track. In addition, they can offer alternatives for dealing with the situation.

Following are some suggestions for introducing and executing a managed change process:

1. Start with a clear mission, a short list of core corporate values, and a well-defined vision.

2. Let followers know that leadership wants to work with them in creating a strong corporate culture based on the organization's mission, values, and vision. They need to know that they are critical to the success of the undertaking.

3. Explain that while building a more effective organization is the primary focus, change must also occur within the individual. Remind followers that they must all take a fresh look at their actions, values, and perceptions.

4. Solicit feedback on your leadership style. Some typical questions might be, "How is my behavior being received?" "How should I modify my behavior?" "What should I do differently, how should I do it, and why would a new approach be more successful?"

5. Prepare the leadership team for regression and backsliding. Remind your closest associates and subordinates that managed change is evolutionary and that a certain amount of regression and backsliding are inevitable.

6. Suggest that members of the leadership team make themselves psychologically bulletproof. Ask them to remain objective and focused on the vision and to take care not to personalize any issues. In turn, suggest that they respond to any backsliding on your part with, "I don't appreciate your behavior, but I'll do what you tell me to do because we're in this together."

In moving through the change process, remember that one person alone cannot produce change. A conductor produces no music without the orchestra; a football coach is not on the field with the players. All members of the team must be willing to change. Nevertheless, wanting change is a good beginning but not enough to effect that change, nor is a well-written action plan. Within the organization, four or five individuals may lack the values, skills, or knowledge to help the organization become more effective. Perhaps some of these individuals will be able to make the necessary adjustments, but others will inevitably leave. If the decision is that the orchestra will no longer play Sousa marches but progressive jazz, this will be bad news for the sousaphone player!

The myths of change discussed above can easily be debunked by a simple description and even simpler concept of all humans and change. Figure 2.1 shows the continuum from enthusiastic change to massive resistance. The underlying concept is that we all change all of the time when the following three conditions are in place:

"No amount of building, visioning, or money can replace the loyalty and commitment of those who work in your organization. Loyalty is earned by deeds and a solid commitment to do the right thing. I would argue that it takes a combination of good coaching and talented athletes' attention to make a winning team. Very few games are won by the coaches or the athletes alone."

—*Richard C. Breon, FACHE, president and CEO, Spectrum Health, Grand Rapids, Michigan*

1. We want the change to happen.
2. We understand why the change is happening.
3. We control the process of the change.

Figure 2.1 reflects the idea that change is easy when the person responsible wants it to happen and controls its process. When people do not want to change (do not understand it) and have no control of the process, they resist aggressively.

Another facet of this dynamic is the fact that happy people resist change because they like the way things are currently, and angry people resist change because they do not want the person

Figure 2.1: The Easy-to-Hard Continuum

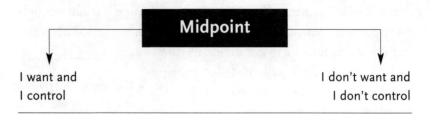

| Midpoint |

I want and
I control

I don't want and
I don't control

driving change to "win." Recognizing this difference is important to the leader who wants a smooth transition.

One final, and very widely held, myth about change needs to be exposed. This is the myth that satisfied employees produce satisfied customers. The fact is that happy employees do not change, because they like the way things are presently. Figure 2.2 shows the midpoint or area of change, sometimes called "cognitive dissonance or cognitive disequilibrium." Change does not happen at the extremes of this continuum. Only when the world seems a little uncomfortable do people change. When the world is in stasis and the group targeted to change is content, there is no imperative to change. When the group targeted to change is angry, it also will not change, whether or not the change is imperative.

My first article on the myths of employee satisfaction was published in the March/April 1999 issue of *Healthcare Executive*. The main thrust of the article is encapsulated by the following excerpt: "While satisfied employees are content with the way things are, motivated employees work toward the way things will be. To remain satisfied, employees need their satisfiers to be continually renewed; to remain motivated, employees work to find new and interesting challenges. Shift your focus from employee satisfaction to employee motivation if you want your organization to truly succeed" (Atchison 1999, 23).

This notion was not universally accepted in the healthcare field at the time mainly because it ran counter to decades of titled

Figure 2.2: The Anxiety/Behavior Continuum

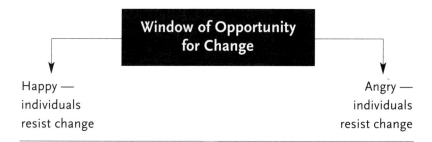

healthcare executives and human resources professionals spending many millions of dollars on "happiness scales" for their employees. The strong pushback triggered by the first article led me to write a second article (Atchison 2003) on the myths of employee satisfaction in 2003. Figure 2.3 shows a more in-depth treatment of the sources of employee satisfaction.

Satisfaction has two sources. The first source is something *given* to you that makes you happy. The second source is something *earned* that produces the feeling of satisfaction from prideful work.

In essence, then, the ability of an employee to become a follower is a function of the skill of the leader to create a workplace (an ecosystem) that promotes pride, loyalty, and ownership—the critical qualities of commitment. Building commitment to the organization's change process is the defining characteristic of a successful healthcare leader. Leaders understand and consistently demonstrate the ten most important ways to build commitment to a change process:

1. Involve or engage all of the people who will be affected by a program or system.
2. Create a "no fault transfer" norm in which everyone loses when one loses.
3. Negotiate win-win solutions. Success is defined by how many individuals succeed.

Figure 2.3: The Satisfaction/Pride Continuum

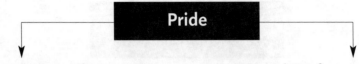

Egocentric Satisfaction	Other-Centered Satisfaction
What have you done for me lately?	How can I help you?
Satisfaction results from external, episodic, short-term, noncontingent pleasantness.	Satisfaction results from prideful and meaningful work. The source of the satisfaction is internal, long lasting, and contingent on performance.
Example: Finding a good parking spot or getting a free dessert on your birthday	Example: Finishing a four-year degree while working full-time or helping someone in need

4. Use goal clarity to focus each follower on the critical task that is derived directly from the corporate mission.
5. Emphasize the dynamics of change, mainly that there are no quick fixes. Be flexible throughout the process, because change will continue to accelerate at an unpredictable rate.
6. Focus on the human components (the intangibles) of quality, achievement, and profitability.
7. Use data to promote commitment—Dx precedes Rx.
8. Adapt managed change strategies throughout the organization based on the unique characteristics of the group. For example, postoperative nurses have different needs than staff in the dietary and accounts payable departments. One size cannot fit all.
9. Write a positive vision of the organization's future. Look at problems as challenges and opportunities, and be proactive.

10. Nurture a sense of teamwork. Followers who share the same goal and understand their role interdependency are much more successful than employees who work in "silos."

Some employees will never engage in a managed change process. There is a group of workers, typically called cynics, who will never follow. For whatever reason, these workers get more gratification out of sabotaging and discrediting a change process than out of organizational improvement. The simple question differentiating followers and cynics is, how much are you willing to commit to the success of our organization? Fortunately, cynics usually comprise only 1 to 3 percent of the workforce. Despite their small number, however, they can be very noisy and toxic to success, and they must be replaced. It is impossible to maximize followership when cynics are allowed to stay.

> "One of the first items of business when I visit a hospital is to ensure that the mission statement is a true reflection of the actual operations and that the hospital's mission is widely known and understood by employees at all levels."
>
> —Michael Rust, FACHE, president and CEO, Kentucky Hospital Association, Louisville, Kentucky

CONCLUSION

Change is possible. Managing change is what leaders do. Leaders have followers who commit to the mission and share the vision for the future. Several myths, if believed, can interfere with the ability of a titled executive to maximize the achievement of the organization. The most damaging myth deals with the titled executive's inability or unwillingness to create a strong corporate culture anchored in a powerful mission statement.

Other significant myths deal with human motivation. The main question this book attempts to answer is, why do workers follow leaders? To a lesser degree, this book considers why some titled healthcare executives never have followers. The easiest way to understand why some staff are motivated to follow while others seem to be motivated not to follow is to remember that motivation is a function of meaning: We are all motivated to display those behaviors that have the most meaning to us. Leaders are able to create a work environment that aligns the values of the workers with the corporate values and allows the workers to see how they contribute to the mission.

Leaders know that the key that unlocks followership is commitment. Commitment is the combination of pride and loyalty to the organization as well as a feeling of ownership in those decisions that most affect them. Without commitment, your followership is nothing but an illusion.

REFERENCES

Atchison, T. 1999. "The Myths of Employee Satisfaction." *Healthcare Executive* 14 (2): 18–23.

———. 2003. "Exposing the Myths of Employee Satisfaction." Healthcare Executive 18 (3): 20–26.

Lundin, S. C., H. Paul, and J. Christensen. 2000. *Fish! A Remarkable Way to Boost Morale and Improve Results*. New York: Hyperion Books.

Reinertsen, J. 1999. Presentation, VHA Mountain States Meeting, Keystone, CO.

Watson, T. J. 1963. *A Business and Its Beliefs: The Ideas that Helped Build IBM*. New York: McGraw-Hill.

CHAPTER 3

Perspectives on Increasing Followership

FOLLOWERSHIP IS DIFFICULT to achieve. Not everyone can create followers; leaders somehow inspire followers, whereas titled executives try to manage behavior in an effort to make followers out of subordinates. *Modern Healthcare's* Chuck Lauer, HFACHE, in one of his many thoughtful "Publisher's Letters," states that "People want someone to mentor and inspire them, not micromanage their every action and second-guess them when they do their jobs" (Lauer 2003) No one as yet has adequately explained why this difference exists between leaders who inspire and managers who control—is it genetic, environmental, situational, learned, or some combination of these factors? Some call this difference the "X factor," which seems to be a scholarly attempt at disguising the fact that we do not know why some have followers and some never will.

While the etiology of leadership remains a mystery, the characteristics that attract followers are widely understood. Many leadership characteristics can be learned; however, the ability to use these tools to create followers is unique to the individual and the situation. For example, Tiger Woods's golf coach could teach any of us the same things he teaches Tiger. However, knowing the mechanics behind Tiger's play does not mean that we can execute the process with his skills. The same phenomenon exists with leadership development: knowing the characteristics of the world's greatest leaders does not guarantee followers.

LEADERSHIP MODELS

While the X factor will always lie mysteriously in the art of followership, there is a science to leadership that can be taught, and this science has several useful models. These models describe why some executives have followers (i.e., leaders) and some executives do not have followers (i.e., titled executives).

Multidimensional Model

Jim Collins's (2001) research-based book, *Good to Great: Why Some Companies Make the Leap . . . and Others Don't*,* uses a multidimensional model based on three domains: disciplined people, disciplined thought, and disciplined action. Collins believes that successful leaders, or "disciplined people," possess unique characteristics that make up "level 5 leadership." This status is displayed by ". . . a paradoxical mix of personal humility and professional will. They are ambitious, to be sure, but ambitious first and foremost for the company, not themselves" (39). Disciplined people also exhibit the "first who . . . then what" concept. Leaders who are able to generate the most followers went through the following sequence: "they *first* got the right people on the bus (and the wrong people off the bus) and then figured out where to drive it" (41).

Collins's second domain of successful leaders is "disciplined thought," which includes the "confront the brutal facts" and "hedgehog" concepts. The data that Collins gathered from great companies related to the "brutal facts" idea reveal that "Leadership

---

* Material from *Good to Great: Why Some Companies Make the Leap . . . and Others Don't* by Jim Collins. Copyright © 2001 by Jim Collins. Reprinted with permission from Jim Collins and HarperCollins Publishers Inc.

does not begin with just vision. It begins with getting people to confront the brutal facts and to act on the implementations" (89). The hedgehog concept is stated very simply as follows: "Hedgehogs see the essential and ignore the rest" (91).

The last domain Collins discusses is "disciplined action," which includes a "culture of discipline" and "technology accelerators." A culture of discipline refers to a duality: "On the one hand, it requires people who adhere to a consistent system; yet, on the other hand, it gives people freedom and responsibility within the framework of that system" (142). The notion of technology accelerators means that great companies ". . . avoid technology fads and bandwagons, yet they become pioneers in the application of carefully selected technologies" (162).

Jim Collins does an excellent job of describing a model in which followers thrive. He lists the critical leadership characteristics and shows how these traits create an ecosystem, or workplace environment, that underpins and sustains business success through the right people. The main ingredients in moving from good to great are, according to Collins, focus and discipline.

Military Model

One leadership model that has stood the test of time is that of the military. Colonel Dandridge M. Malone (Ret.) (1983)† is the author of a well-written book about the way ". . . you get the men in your unit to do what you say." Malone lists the 16 leadership behaviors every leader needs to display.

1. Courage, demonstrated by taking risks and acting calmly and firmly in stressful situations.

---

† From SMALL UNIT LEADERSHIP by Dandridge M. Malone, copyright © 1983 by Dandridge M. Malone. Used by permission of Presidio Press, an imprint of The Ballantine Publishing Group, a division of Random House, Inc.

2. Bearing, demonstrated by setting and maintaining high standards of appearance.
3. Decisiveness, demonstrated by studying your decisions and carefully selecting the best course of action, and knowing when not to make a decision.
4. Dependability, demonstrated by being at places on time when you are told to be there or when you say you will.
5. Endurance, demonstrated by maintaining the physical and mental stamina to perform your duties under stress conditions for extended periods of time.
6. Enthusiasm, demonstrated by consistently communicating a positive attitude.
7. Humility, demonstrated by describing your unit's performance in terms of "what we did" not "what I did."
8. Humor, demonstrated by having fun on your job.
9. Initiative, demonstrated by looking for and figuring out better ways to do things.
10. Integrity, demonstrated by telling the truth and encouraging honest and open communication.
11. Judgment, demonstrated by closely considering a range of alternatives before you act.
12. Justice, demonstrated by making decisions that support mission accomplishment and listening to all sides of an issue before making a decision.
13. Knowledge, demonstrated by making sound tactical decisions.
14. Tact, demonstrated by speaking to others with the same kind of respect you expect yourself.
15. Loyalty, demonstrated by passing on and carrying out tough orders of superiors without expressing personal criticism.
16. Selflessness, demonstrated by ensuring that the needs of your soldiers are met before attending to your own needs.

Secretary of State General Colin Powell (Ret.) enjoys an international reputation as a great leader. People believe him, trust him, and follow him. In "Quotations from Powell: A Leadership Primer," the appendix to Oren Harari's (2002, 27–29) book *The Leadership Secrets of Colin Powell*,‡ Secretary of State Powell provides 18 lessons in leadership. These lessons support his belief that "Leadership is the art of accomplishing more than the science of management says is possible." The 18 lessons are reprinted below.

> "Gaining organizational commitment is the most undervalued and misunderstood need that healthcare organizations have today. Healthcare systems will not succeed without leadership that understands and has mastered this skill."
>
> —Samuel L. Odle, FACHE, senior vice president and COO, Methodist Hospital of Indiana, Indianapolis

1. Being responsible sometimes means pissing people off.
2. The day soldiers stop bringing you their problems is the day you have stopped leading them. They have either lost confidence that you can help them or concluded that you do not care. Either case is a failure of leadership.
3. Don't be buffaloed by experts and elites. Experts often possess more data than judgment.
4. Don't be afraid to challenge the pros, even in their own backyard.
5. Never neglect the details. When everyone's mind is dulled or distracted the leader must be doubly vigilant.
6. You don't know what you can get away with until you try.
7. Keep looking below surface appearances. Don't shrink from doing so [just] because you might not like what you find.
8. Organizations don't really accomplish anything. Plans don't accomplish anything, either. Theories of management don't much matter. Endeavors succeed or fail because of the people involved. Only by attracting the best people will you accomplish great deeds.

---

‡ From O. Harari, THE LEADERSHIP SECRETS OF COLIN POWELL, copyright © 2002, McGraw-Hill. Material reproduced with permission of The McGraw-Hill Companies.

9. Organization charts and fancy titles count for next to nothing.

10. Never let your ego get so close to your position that when your position goes, your ego goes with it.

11. Fit no stereotypes. Don't chase the latest management fads. The situation dictates which approach best accomplishes the team's mission.

12. Perpetual optimism is a force multiplier.

13. Powell's Rules for Picking People: Look for intelligence and judgment, and most critically, a capacity to anticipate, to see around corners. Also, look for loyalty, integrity, a high energy drive, a balanced ego, and the drive to get things done.

14. Great leaders are almost always great simplifiers, who can cut through argument, debate and doubt, to offer a solution everyone can understand.

15. Part I: Use the formula $P = 40$ to 70, in which P stands for the probability of success and the numbers indicate the percentage of information acquired. Part II: Once the information is in the 40 to 70 range, go with your gut.

16. The commander in the field is always right and the rear echelon is wrong, unless proven otherwise.

17. Have fun in your command. Don't always run at a breakneck pace. Take leave when you've earned it: Spend time with your families. Corollary: Surround yourself with people who take their work seriously, but not themselves, those who work hard and play hard.

18. Command is lonely.

Cohesion/Clarity Obsession Model

Patrick Lencioni (2000, 141) presents his model of creating followers in *The Four Obsessions of an Extraordinary Executive*.§ He

---

§ Material from *The Four Obsessions of an Extraordinary Executive* by Patrick Lencioni. Copyright © 2000, John Wiley & Sons. This material is used by permission of John Wiley & Sons, Inc.

believes that healthy organizations are dominated by inspired followers because the leaders of these organizations obsess about achieving the following four goals:

1. Build and maintain a cohesive leadership team.
2. Create organizational clarity.
3. Overcommunicate organizational clarity.
4. Reinforce organizational clarity through human systems. (141)

Employee Encouragement Model

Another model is presented by Stephen Lundin, Harry Paul, and John Christensen (2000, 78) in the entertaining, amazingly popular, and very short book called *Fish! A Remarkable Way to Boost Morale and Improve Results.*** *Fish!* discusses several principles for creating a work environment that encourages followers. These are summarized below.

- Your attitude sets the tone for your environment. Consider your reactions, frame of mind, and persona as you go through your work day.
- A sense of play is important to creating a setting that supports followership. Think about how you can develop a fun and energized workplace.
- The attitudes of your customers, both internal and external, are a reflection of how you engage them. Do you strive to make their day a good one?
- Being at work is not the same as being present. Be fully involved in every aspect of your job, attending to the small details and the fleeting encounters as well as the high-visibility actions and interactions.

** It fascinates me that we have gone from "moving cheese" to "throwing fish." People are completely retooling large and complicated organizations based on very short books that use food metaphors. Maybe I should end this book with a short description about how creating followers is like making a salad!

Colleague Model

James M. Kouzes and Barry Z. Posner (1993) wrote a very interesting book in which the dynamics of leaders and followers is a major topic. Their book, *Credibility: How Leaders Gain and Lose It, Why People Demand It,*‡ contains a great deal of data about how leaders and followers view each other. They found that "In virtually every survey . . . honesty has always ranked first on all lists. Competence has also received votes from the majority of respondents. . . . We want to know that our leaders and our colleagues are worthy of trust, and we desire that our leaders and our colleagues be capable and effective" (254). However, Kouzes and Posner discovered that while these two characteristics are sought in both leaders and colleagues, leaders separate themselves from colleagues on some very important dimensions. They state that

> We have noted that people expect their leaders to be forward-looking, to have a sense of direction and a concern for the future of the organization. People also expect leaders to be inspiring—to be energetic and positive about the future. Leaders must be able to communicate their visions in ways that uplift and encourage people to enlist. In combination, being forward-looking and inspiring make a leader visionary and dynamic. They make a person attractive to others. They point people in pioneering directions and give them energy and drive. They get people focused on and enthusiastic about building the organization of the future, putting today's actions in a strategic context. Add to this the rest of the foundation of credibility (honesty and competence) and you would think you would have an unbeatable formula for success. (255)

---

‡ Material from *Credibility: How Leaders Gain and Lose It, Why People Demand It* by James M. Kouzes and Barry Z. Posner. Copyright © 1993, John Wiley & Sons. This material is used by permission of John Wiley & Sons, Inc.

All of these models and lists of characteristics describe those very important individuals who are able to inspire followers. The deeper dimension of each of these models and lists lies in the nature of human motivation.

GAINING ORGANIZATIONAL COMMITMENT

Understanding Motivation

To become a better leader, you must first understand a few basic principles of human motivation—specifically, you must understand what motivates people to work. Psychodynamic, developmental, biophysical, and behavioral theories are useful in explaining many kinds of human behavior. However, they are not the best models to explain leadership and organizational behavior. Let us turn instead to Martin Maehr and Larry Braskamp's (1986) *The Motivation Factor: A Theory of Personal Investment.* Their book quite simply looks at motivation from the standpoint of how people spend their time, talent, and energy. Consider your own behavior. How do you spend your time? When you get a series of phone calls, in what order do you return them? Of even more significance, whom do you call at noon or 5:00 p.m. because you know they probably will not be in their office? In contrast, whom do you call right away?

We frequently exhibit conflicts between our words and our actions. In fact, the biggest problem that we have as healthcare

> "Commitment is situational. For example, in a crisis (emergency room or battlefield), gaining the commitment of followers is often less difficult as they quickly realize the immediacy of the situation. However, when there is no crisis, obtaining followership is more difficult. There seems to be two factors that create followers in a noncrisis situation: (1) the leader's ability to make good decisions and (2) a clear demonstration that the leader cares about the individuals he/she wants as followers."
>
> —CAPT Anthony Sebbio, MSC, USN, CHE

professionals is that many times *we lie to ourselves.* The following scenarios provide examples:

- A titled executive claims he is caring, sensitive, and compassionate, but he spends six months a year worrying about his hospital's budget and another six months defending it. Where does the truth lie?
- A financial manager reports the net operating margin to three decimal points but has no sense of her organization's core values. She pays lip service to care for the poor but offers only a 2 percent write-off as evidence of her concern. If this titled executive really wanted to care for the poor, would she not invest more of her time, talent, and energy in doing so?
- In speeches and annual reports, a titled executive may speak often and eloquently of the quality of care offered by the institution. However, the nurses confide to colleagues, "We're pressured to make money; we're a profit center." Behavior and motivation are driven solely by the organization's desire to safeguard its economic position.

To know why people follow, watch how they spend their time, talent, and energy. To know what they value most, take a look at task perseverance. Followers stay with tasks that meet their criteria for motivation, but they procrastinate when the task fails to "turn them on." If a manager takes only a week to write a proposal for a new marketing program but consistently submits her variance reports a month late, she provides a fairly clear notion of what makes her tick. Good intentions and well-meaning words are not behavior; talking is not doing. Claiming to be motivated to do something serves no purpose if the person does not persevere at the behavior. What does it matter if an administrative assistant claims he is working hard but makes 15 personal calls per day, fails to come in on time, takes long lunches, and consistently leaves early?

To inspire followers today, you must learn to focus on the frequency and duration of employees' behaviors if you want to determine what drives and motivates them. As an exercise, observe two or three managers or employees for two weeks. Watch what they do and how often they do it as well as how long a given behavior lasts. Assessing what it would take to change their behavior will give you a fairly clear idea of the strength of their motivation—that is, where they are investing their time, talent, and energy.

Four Key Values

Ultimately, the motivation to invest personally in work lies in the relationship of personal values to corporate values. In *The Motivation Factor*, Maehr and Braskamp outline four values that shape personal investment: (1) recognition, (2) accomplishment, (3) power, and (4) affiliation. Recognition and accomplishment deal with how staff members relate to work, job, task, or activity, and power and affiliation pertain to people, relationships, friends, and colleagues.

Recognition. Some followers crave attention. They continually seek feedback on the quality of their work from their bosses and colleagues. To be seen as high-producing winners is all-important to them. They enjoy seeing their name in print, winning awards, and receiving public recognition at special events. For these followers, the emphasis is on external reinforcement of good work through verbal and written plaudits, awards, perks, supplemental benefits, and merit and salary increases.

Accomplishment. In their offices by 7:30 a.m., some followers race through project after project. They are eager to get involved in new ventures in the hope of achieving ever greater things. Anchored to their desks, these followers rarely take time out for lunch or routine conversation. In their professional life they emphasize productivity, doing the job right, and exploring new opportunities.

Power. Some followers just want to win. They enjoy going head-to-head with the president of the medical staff, the chairperson of the city planning council, and anyone else they encounter. Instead of feeling intimidated by escalating competition from neighboring hospitals, they are exhilarated by it. Their professional life is driven by competition and conflict and the quest for power and position.

Affiliation. Finally, some followers want to create a family feeling among their fellow staff members. They invest at least one-third of their day trying to build an atmosphere of trust and camaraderie among all the employees. Birthdays, anniversaries, graduations, and births are celebrated with lunches and receptions. When an employee has a personal or family problem, they take time to talk it through with him or her and suggest solutions. Their professional life is driven by a desire to care for and respect other employees and to treat them as part of the hospital family.

Everyone is motivated by these four needs, but to varying degrees. Among executives, power tends to be the dominant value; however, the percentages of other values can shift as a result of circumstances. For example, the need for recognition might accelerate when a person feels threatened, and the value of accomplishment might jump dramatically during a budget crunch. But even if the values of recognition and accomplishment expand at times, they will always be subordinate to the dominant motivational value of power.

Typical Patterns

Do typical values patterns apply to different types of professions? Viewed from the standpoint of *The Motivation Factor*, Maehr and Braskamp indicate that the typical healthcare professional is high in affiliation, medium high in power, and medium in recognition and accomplishment. A salesperson, in contrast, tends to be high in accomplishment, recognition, and power but low in affiliation.

A successful healthcare leader is typically medium in power and recognition and high in accomplishment and affiliation.

Emphasizing one value rather than another is not good or bad in itself. The problem begins when conflict occurs between the values that employees have and the kinds of values that the organization needs. For example, strategic plans often emphasize high recognition, accomplishment, and power values. But these plans would stand a greater chance for success if they were built on high accomplishment, medium power and affiliation, and medium to low recognition. The point is that leaders intuitively recognize that the value structures of the followers and the organization may differ. Leaders accept those differences and work to build strong cultures that align organizational values with followers' personal values.

When a personal value system fails to align with job expectations and the organization's core values, serious problems may result. For example, after 30 years in Catholic healthcare, a member of a religious order will likely have too many conflicting values if asked to run a for-profit subsidiary. In the same way, a hard-driving MBA may have little patience with extended dialogs on the need for compassionate care.

Matching personal with organizational values is the most critical challenge of creating followers. The difficulty here, of course, is that each individual sees the world through his or her own eyes. A marketing vice president with the dominant value of accomplishment has trouble seeing why her staff likes to adjourn a half hour early on Friday afternoons and go out for a drink or why her secretary resents receiving a stack of written directives at 4:00 p.m. In the same way, a hospice director whose dominant value is affiliation may view her power-driven, numbers-focused vice president of professional services as unfeeling. Or nurses who have given their lives to caring for patients and their families may have difficulty relating to physicians driven by power and accomplishment.

Does this mean that leaders should surround themselves with colleagues and subordinates who share the same dominant work values? No. If an affiliation-oriented human resources director hires staff who are exclusively driven by affiliation, the human resources function will probably suffer. People will spend so much time socializing with each other that nothing will get done. Although a group of highly affiliative nurses can usually work well together, a highly affiliative senior management group might run an institution into the ground in a few years. In the same way, a heavy-hitting, power-oriented chief information officer might lock horns and do battle with a data processing manager for whom power is an equally strong value. In such cases, one can only hope that a third party will emerge to coax the power-driven executives into opposite corners and refocus the combatants on their roles in achieving the organization's vision. Otherwise, the urge to dominate, compete, control, and win may come to obsess them.

Leaders, then, surround themselves with diverse people. On an intuitive level, they understand dominant values and motivational drives and choose people who complement their style. William Foley, FACHE, president and CEO of Provena Health in Mokena, Illinois, built an effective team from widely diverse and exceptionally competent professionals. Understanding the values of recognition, accomplishment, power, and affiliation helped Foley to comprehend the dynamics of his team. His ability to focus such an intelligent and high-energy group demonstrates his leadership and explains his organization's success. He followed Collins's notion, "First get the right people on the bus."

If a person views himself as a power-oriented executive who is more likely to persevere at a task for the sake of winning rather than out of relish for the task itself, he should put together a team of people who rank high on the values of recognition, affiliation, and accomplishment. He should find people who can work hard and who will commit themselves to the vision and be loyal to the organization.

Keep in mind that power is not by itself a negative. Leadership is power used positively. The power of leadership is defined not by what you say or believe but by the followers who are willing to stand behind you. If a titled executive declares, "We're going to move in this direction," and staff says, "You're nuts," that executive may have authority, but he is not a leader. Power only comes from his title, not his followers.

In the final analysis, leaders need to understand and manage all four values. Consider the analogy of the human body. To have a body that is all heart, muscle, brain, or nervous system would be dysfunctional. A human being needs all these organs and systems. In the same way, an organization needs a balance of the values of accomplishment (the head), affiliation (the heart), power (the muscular system), and recognition (the nervous system). Truly outstanding leaders, such as Foley, understand the interactive dynamics of these values and can balance them in such a way as to put the *right person* in the *right job* in the *right corporate culture.*

> "Getting commitment only happens in an open and trusting environment."
>
> —*Wayne Lerner,* DR.P.H., FACHE, *president and* CEO, *Rehabilitation Institute of Chicago*

Let us next examine each of these values and see how they are expressed in terms of a corporate culture.

VALUES IN THE ENVIRONMENT

Many people invest a great deal of time and money to present themselves in certain ways. Ambience and environment offer clues to a leader's dominant values and expectations of others. This section and those that follow highlight some examples of each value set.

Recognition. Is there an office shrine filled with plaques and autographed photos taken with political leaders and other celebrities? This executive craves attention, and you can motivate her by recognizing and praising her performance.

Accomplishment. Does this executive's office feature halogen lights, a fax machine, a personal digital assistant, worksheets, and a laptop computer in addition to a desktop PC? Offer this executive well-edited data and information at a brisk pace. Time is this leader's currency.

Power. Is this executive's office dominated by an enormous mahogany desk, a credenza, and a conference table in perfect condition? Expect power-driven responses. Does the bookshelf contain a few select awards and national best sellers on executive leadership? This person is a competitor, someone who wants to win and who enjoys gaining authority and control over others. Be prepared for some tough verbal jousting.

Affiliation. Is this executive's office immaculate and decorated simply in soft, muted tones? Are fresh flowers and other pleasing artifacts displayed prominently? This leader rises from his desk to greet you and asks how you are feeling. In working with this person, expect him to place emphasis on building a team and to go out of his way to help others on the team.

VALUES IN EVALUATION

Performance evaluations show clearly the dominant work values of the evaluator. Many times, in fact, the evaluation process shows more about the evaluator than the one being evaluated.

Recognition. The titled executive motivated by recognition wants to believe that an employee's successful performance is a direct result of the executive's strong leadership. His evaluation of an employee might sound like this: "*I'm* really concerned about how you feel about this evaluation and your work here at Health, Inc. *I'd* like to spend some time discussing how I can help you even more in the years to come. *I've* noticed that you've really thrived since you transferred into *my* division a year ago. *I* think you'll agree that *I've* really done a great job in developing some of your outstanding skills and talents. *I'm* really pleased you were able to mesh with *me* and produce such dramatic results for *my* hospital. You've really grown under *my* leadership."

Power. The power-oriented executive tends to challenge an employee's behavior and often suggests that the employee emulate her style. An evaluation typically goes like this: "The way you handled those community clinic joint ventures showed some inconsistencies in judgment. If you look back at how the CT scanner was handled, you'll get a better idea of where you could have gained an edge. You could have questioned harder and received more concessions. We play hardball here, and next year you need to stiffen your spine and tough out better negotiations. You've got the right talent and education, but you need to push harder because next year is going to be even tougher than this year. You did all right this year, but we're in this game to win over the long haul. There are only Ws (winners) and Ls (losers)—if you behave like an L, you're history!"

Affiliation. The affiliation-oriented executive openly shares information and shows care and concern for the employee's welfare. He would begin an evaluation this way: "How are you feeling today? Well, it looks like it's time for your evaluation again; I hope this is a good day for you. Before we sit down and talk, why don't you take some time and review the evaluation form I've completed? We'll probably need quite a bit of time to discuss this, so why don't you clear your calendar for the rest of the day? I don't think there's anything in here that's going to upset you, but I know this is really important to you, and I want this to be a positive experience. Now, if it's not helpful, I want you to please tell me. You know you can talk to me. I think you know how I feel about your being with us and how much you've helped us all."

Accomplishment. The executive who is accomplishment oriented sees success as a matter of meeting corporate objectives. Her fast-

> "Creating followers is easy as long as we remember the essence of the human condition—which is, the need to matter and the need to be needed." [Paraphrased from Viktor Frankl in the conclusion to *Man's Search for Meaning* (New York: Washington Square Press, 1997].
>
> —*Joseph S. Bujak*, M.D., *vice president of medical affairs, Kootenai Medical Center, Coeur d'Alene, Idaho*

moving, staccato evaluations often leave employees breathless: "OK, you met your department's first five strategic objectives, but you're still working on those last two. Let's look at next year. I think we've got some fairly strong criteria. I've got to tell you, you've got a bunch of people over there, but you don't have a team, you know what I mean? You've got some real all-stars, but I don't see them working together. You know what I'm saying? Now, I want to see real force there next year. Let's get all that energy moving in one direction. It's not there yet. When will it happen?"

VALUES IN DECISION MAKING

Executives with certain value profiles also have unique ways of making decisions.

Power. The power-oriented executive may create a facade of participation, involvement, and consensus, but the decision she wants has already been made. Her skill is in getting others to buy into that decision and in taking control of implementation. When she makes a decision, she sticks with it. To do otherwise is to "lose."

Recognition. The recognition-oriented executive takes credit for decisions. He gives special emphasis to how he personally resolved conflicts, involved others, and gathered information during the arduous decision-making process. According to his account, there would have been no decision if it were not for his outstanding skills in negotiation, problem solving, and consensus building. All he craves is recognition as the team's savior and spiritual guide. "See what I did for you. Yet again, I showed you how important I am."

Affiliation. The affiliation-dominated executive often has problems making decisions. He goes out of his way to ensure that

> "There are three leadership principles that encourage followship (both in the military and civilian life). They are: (1) always accomplish the mission, (2) ensure the welfare of your troops, and (3) set the example."
>
> —COL *Allen Gildersleeve, MSC, U.S. Army (Ret.)*

everyone contributes to and feels good about a decision. Because he feels compelled to seek continual feedback from others, he hesitates to announce a final decision. If a decision is made quickly, he worries that he may not have gotten everyone's input. In the worst case, he will sacrifice a decision. If a power-oriented colleague declares, "I don't want to do that. I've got a better idea," he may respond, "OK, that sounds like a good idea."

Accomplishment. The accomplishment-oriented executive wants data and action—and she wants it now. She sweeps people into action by urging them to clear their calendars so that they can get together and hammer out a plan. She quickly mobilizes all the resources—from outside consultants to off-site retreat locations—that will be needed to get the job done. Echoing themes of innovation, challenge, and opportunity, she decides quickly and has little patience for people who do not understand the need to move ahead rapidly.

CONCLUSION

The science of leadership has been developed and refined over the centuries. The more elusive art of leadership continues to be the X factor. The same leadership skills will not work with all followers. Regardless of the leadership behaviors displayed, the X factor seems to be the ability to have followers perceive competency, intensity, consistency, courage, and humility. The X factor is that followers trust the leader.

REFERENCES

Collins, J. 2001. *Good to Great: Why Some Companies Make the Leap . . . and Others Don't.* New York: HarperCollins.

Harari, O. 2002. *The Leadership Secrets of Colin Powell.* New York: McGraw-Hill.

Kouzes, J. M., and B. Posner. 1993. *Credibility: How Leaders Gain and Lose It, Why People Demand It*. San Francisco: Jossey-Bass.

Lauer, C. 2003. "Publisher's Letter." *Modern Healthcare* Jan. 6: 25.

Lencioni, P. 2000. *The Four Obsessions of an Extraordinary Executive*. San Francisco: Jossey-Bass.

Lundin, S. C., H. Paul, and J. Christensen. 2000. *Fish! A Remarkable Way to Boost Morale and Improve Results*. New York: Hyperion Books.

Maehr, M., and L. Braskamp. 1986. *The Motivation Factor: A Theory of Personal Investment*. Lanham, MD: Lexington Books.

Malone, D. M. 1983. *Small Unit Leadership: A Commonsense Approach*. Novato, CA: Presidio Press.

CHAPTER 4

Ensuring Motivated Employees: Lessons from Healthcare

ALL HEALTHCARE ORGANIZATIONS have three parts: the personalities of the individuals who comprise the workforce, the specific characteristics and expectations for the "job," and the ecosystem or work environment (i.e., corporate culture) in which work is carried out.

The previous chapter presented several models and lists of characteristics describing how leaders inspire followers. Regardless of whether the thoughts came from the head of the Joint Chiefs of Staff or a Seattle fish store, the models and lists have many overlapping notions. The essential factors of effective leaders seem to be a constant demonstration that the followers are (1) cared for and (2) cared about. The by-product of such caring is a degree of trust of followers that differentiates the leader from the titled executive. This chapter builds on these models and lists by presenting healthcare data from organizations with titled executives and case studies of organizations in which the leaders have a lot of followers. All of the leadership cases are instructive because of how they aligned the three parts of any successful healthcare organization—people, job, and culture.

HEALTHCARE'S CURRENT STATE OF PEOPLE, JOB, AND CULTURE

During one of the initial focus groups of a recently merged health-care system, a nurse manager described her current work environment as "the negative vortex of doom." This statement describes a work environment that reinforces negativity over positive thoughts and negative comments over productive work. In fact, in the polluted, toxic subcultures to which this statement refers a badge of honor seems to be awarded to whoever can be the most negative. Attempts at "one-upsmanship" are replaced by "one-downsmanship."

This example is not an isolated occurrence. The following comments are an amalgamation of several dozen interviews of professional healthcare workers (including physicians) in management positions or higher. These interviews were completed in 2002 and 2003 and were requested to determine the degree of toxicity in the various subgroups. All of the organizations participating in the surveys had recently gone through a leadership transition from a titled executive who focused mainly on the tangibles (especially the finances) to someone who wanted to inspire followers. The most frequently expressed perceptions are discussed in the sections below.

Expressions Reflecting a Toxic Environment

1. We are out of control.
2. We experience enormous time pressures.
3. No clear priorities are set.
4. Support from our bosses and peers is lacking.
5. I am often blindsided by decisions, and as a result I feel incompetent.
6. I am angry and bitter.

7. I keep working faster, but I know I will never catch up.
8. Work takes too much of my time away from my family.
9. Assignment of roles is extremely confusing.
10. We encounter too much blame and not enough rewards.

This list could go on for pages. These ten were selected because they represent the majority of toxic issues healthcare professionals currently experience with titled executives.

Expressions Reflecting Inspiring Leadership

Another way to view the same problem in today's healthcare industry is to list the answers to the core question of this book: What do healthcare leaders do to inspire you to follow?

1. Demonstrate credibility, trust, and respect.
2. Always display ethical and professional behavior.
3. Show a willingness to resolve conflicts fairly.
4. Establish a clear vision and expectations.
5. Foster human imagination—help us grow.
6. Exude optimism and lead by example.
7. Facilitate collaboration.
8. Recognize and reward employee contributions.
9. Overcommunicate.
10. Encourage fun.

What Followers Desire from Leaders

Most organizational toxins are created in the absence of the following five considerations for employees:

1. Respect
2. Control of the decisions that most affect me

3. Rewards and recognition
4. Balance of life—colleagues and family, job and home, work and play
5. Professional development

Working with the Survey Results

From these interview data, I constructed a new paradigm with a symbolic acronym: FUN. The letters can stand for *fear, uncertainty,* and *negativism,* or they can stand for *focus, understanding,* and *neighborliness.* The two sets of words can be viewed in terms of a continuum for assessing followership within your organization.

Fear   *Focus*
0 points . . . . 10 points

Uncertainty   *Understanding*
0 points . . . . 10 points

Negativism   *Neighborliness*
0 points . . . . 10 points

You may wish to assess the followership potential in your organization by asking a random sample of 30 percent of the staff (including the most active physicians) to mark where on the continuum they perceive the current work environment. Consider the following as you review the results:

- If the average score falls between 4 and 7, you may want to conduct some focus groups to determine what can be improved.
- If the average score is lower than 4, you have a toxic work environment that needs major intervention.
- If your average score is above 7, identify best practices and communicate and celebrate the employees' contribution to a positive workplace.

An Example of Strong Corporate Culture

Kelly Mather, CEO of Sutter Lakeside Hospital in Lakeport, California, understands the power of communication in building a strong corporate culture. Mather and her coleaders have developed a strong team by clarifying the values-based mission and vision of Sutter Lakeside Hospital. She communicates constantly with all staff both directly through her coleaders and indirectly through "messages and metaphors" placed all over the property. Every communication is set in the context of the culture of Sutter Lakeside Hospital. Most importantly, Mather's behavior is the best proof that she believes what she says. Mather is an excellent leader who has followers because she understands the importance of culture, teamwork, communication, and trust. She is Sutter Lakeside Hospital's best role model.

Mather has many followers. She explains her ability to inspire and align followers by using a "puzzle." Mather's puzzle has five discrete pieces: leadership; communication; environment; fun and recognition; and mission (Figure 4.1).

Mather believes that the centerpiece of all successful organizations is trust in and commitment to the mission, values, and vision. She and her leadership team, in concert with the employees and physicians, work hard on maintaining the four puzzle pieces. Each of these domains has many specific aspects that promote followership, and the constant focus on these puzzle pieces has achieved measurable results in both the tangible (business) factors and the intangible (followership) factors. For example, the change in key intangible leadership indicators from when Mather began the fol-

> "First, followers want someone who is credible. And second, they want someone they can trust. Trust is an outcome of consistency. Followers need to know that the leader is predictable. And finally, the most important factor in creating followers is ethical behavior in everything."
>
> —Raymond A. Graeca, CHE, president and CEO, DuBois Regional Medical Center, DuBois, Pennsylvania

Figure 4.1: Sutter Lakeside Hospital's Five-Piece Puzzle for Creating an Environment of Followership

A. *The Five Pieces of the Puzzle*

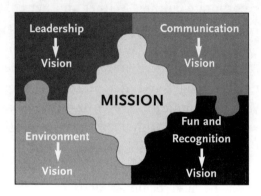

B. *The centerpiece of* SLH's *"puzzle" is the reason it exists—the mission. The four additional puzzle pieces, or steps, are used to keep the mission foremost in mind.*

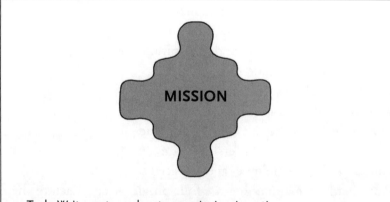

1. Task: Write a story about our mission in action.
2. Discuss story.
3. The most relevant learnings about our corporate culture are . . .
4. Some ways for us to use these learnings are . . .

Figure 4.1 *(continued)*

C. The leadership puzzle piece. Leadership is the first step in SLH's vision achievement. The four steps help leaders learn from each other.

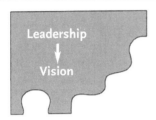

1. Task: Write a story about the importance of leadership at SLH.
2. Discuss story.
3. The most relevant learnings about our corporate culture are . . .
4. Some ways for us to use these learnings are . . .

D. The communication puzzle piece. Communication holds the puzzle pieces together and is the key to building trust. The four steps help clarify what kinds of communication work best to achieve the vision.

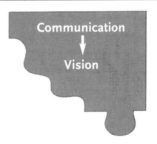

1. Task: Write a story about effective communication.
2. Discuss story.
3. The most relevant learnings about our corporate culture are . . .
4. Some ways for us to use these learnings are . . .

Figure 4.1 *(continued)*

E. The environment puzzle piece. The environment is the ecosystem in which the vision is achieved. The four steps keep the ecosystem free of toxins.

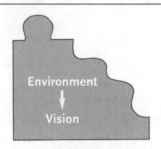

1. Task: Write a story about a positive aspect of our work environment.
2. Discuss story.
3. The most relevant learnings about our corporate culture are . . .
4. Some ways for us to use these learnings are . . .

F. The fun-and-recognition puzzle piece. Fun and recognition reinforce those behaviors that most promote vision achievement. The four steps are used to keep ideas fresh.

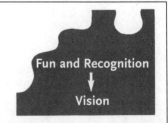

1. Task: Write a story about when you had fun at work.
2. Discuss story.
3. The most relevant learnings about our corporate culture are . . .
4. Some ways for us to use these learnings are . . .

Source: Used with permission of Sutter Lakeside Hospital.

lowership intervention to 12 months later are shown in Table 4.1. The principles that guide Mather are one example of a way to create and sustain followership.

Whether they come to your healthcare organization as nurses, laboratory technicians, or vice presidents, people bring with them a history of personal experience and technical knowledge. The jobs that they perform give them an opportunity to build on their experience and expand their skills while the corporate culture gives them purpose and pride. Leaders must constantly try to fit the right person into the right job within a meaningful culture. When this happens, employees become self-managed, motivated, and productive.

MATCHING PERSONAL AND CORPORATE VALUES

No employee is a *tabula rasa*. When you hire people, you hire their whole history—experiences, skills, and knowledge. A strong leader understands that running an effective organization starts with hiring the right people. The next step is to put these skilled and motivated people into a job where their values and technical skills can flourish. Then the leader continues to build an organizational culture that allows the followers to grow in direct proportion to the organization's success. When the person, job, and organization are moving in the same direction toward a common goal, the organization is effective. But if one element is out of alignment, there is likely to be trouble. A talented and gifted nurse with a rich history of caring can easily get a job in the corporate nursing department of a for-profit multihospital system. Once there, she may find that she enjoys her work but that she dislikes the philosophy of a for-profit system. Her alternatives are to do her job while psychologically disengaging herself from the system, adapt to the new value system, or leave.

Today's situation for nurses is especially poignant. The workforce shortage is real and most likely will get worse as long as toxic work environments are enabled. In years past, hospitals were

Table 4.1: Key Intangible Indicators for the SLH Environment

Assessment	Culture	Job Satisfaction	Commitment
Pre-Intervention	9%	43%	33%
12-Month Assessment	79%	96%	90%

Source: Used with permission of Sutter Lakeside Hospital.

seen as places where patients received care and got well. Today, they may be viewed as costly production lines where very sick people are "fixed" and sent home. Caring clinicians are being forced to embrace industrial engineering productivity models. Many nurses have grown disenchanted because the culture of caring has disappeared from so many hospitals. Whereas a nurse may once have reported to the director of nursing, he now reports to a product-line manager whose goal is to make sure that services contribute to the hospital's business objectives. He may feel comfortable and fulfilled when doing traditional nursing but anxious and resentful when managing a profit center or engaging in cost control and charge capture.

Nurses are facing a conflict between their personal values (why did I enter this profession?), backgrounds, and technical skills as well as a clash between today's economically driven healthcare environment and their own expectations. A person who served the nursing profession for 20 years now finds herself being told, however subtly, that her behavior is somehow wrong or inadequate. If the organization is clumsy about communicating the reasons for necessary changes, it will be increasingly difficult for that nurse to function, no matter how much she likes giving patient care.

Older healthcare executives face a similar dilemma. Those over 40 probably came out of a master's in health administration program in the early 1970s with a heavy dose of history and public health. Their role was to work with trustees on fund development and new building projects and to give physicians whatever they requested. The current numbers-focused MBA mentality runs counter to their experience and education. To cope, a healthcare executive probably depends on one of the three following strategies:

1. *Denial:* "I don't know how to cope with this, but I really don't think the situation is as serious as most people make out. The government will probably tire of this in a few years, and we'll go back to the old system."
    Result: Downward spiral and job loss.
2. *Dependency:* "I don't have the psychological resources to cope with this. I wasn't trained as a cost accountant. I'm going to do what I've always done best and leave this cost stuff to the financial folks."
    Result: Abrogation of significant power to the chief financial officer and possible loss of job.
3. *Leadership:* "Something's happened, but we're going to survive this no matter what it does to other hospitals. We're going to pool our resources and find out what it means for us."
    Result: Inspired people with a new culture that confronts today's challenges and seeks solutions appropriate to the organization. There is a good chance that this leader will thrive regardless of the velocity or volume of change because he has created a team spirit among the workforce that enables it to achieve the vision.

Providing Resources

The ability of an organization to grapple with change by creating followers depends on the amount of meaningful involvement opportunities it creates. If it can help employees see that change is necessary and will produce specific benefits to them, the organization will be able to move forward with inspired followers. As a leader, it is your role to help all followers deal with change. When the next change is considered, look at who will be most threatened by change, and try to understand their dynamics and background. If their values and history conflict with new expectations, work with them. Assure them that while their beliefs and values are still valid, they must now develop new behaviors, such as better record keeping about safety, quality, and costs. Explain how their behavior will help the organization achieve the vision and live the values. Most importantly, support them with staff development that ensures that they have the skills to perform their new tasks.

Leaders must provide the resources to help people change. For example, some systems are writing their own academic curricula for change management. Scripps Health in California, The Methodist Hospital in Texas, Affinity Health System in Wisconsin, Provena Health in Illinois, and Greater Baltimore Medical Center in Maryland are a few examples. Clinical supervisors who rose from the ranks of practioners often end up performing clinical supervisory and leadership functions because that is what today's healthcare requires. However, many are unable to delegate authority or control or manage conflict because they never learned how. Managing change can be learned, but this means acquiring new skills and practicing them. Leaders are successful in moving organizations in new directions because they offer programs that support and inspire followers.

> "Followers hope that the leader is someone they can be loyal to. They want the leader to be competent as a professional and a worthwhile human being."
>
> —Celia Michael, PH.D., administrative director of mental health, New Mexico VA Healthcare System, Albuquerque

Does this mean that everyone can learn how to work in a new environment? No; some employees will not make it. Although every worker deserves an opportunity, change is more difficult for some people than for others. Updating old skills and building new ones can be difficult, and almost impossible, in people who have rigid behaviors. Staff who lead verbal assaults with statements such as, "In my last job, we didn't do it that way"; "We've never done it this way before"; and "It won't work; we tried it ten years ago" may never come around to the new way of doing things. Leaders must wish them the best but remove them compassionately because they do not fit and will never follow.

In the same way, a skilled and valued chief financial officer (CFO) with an authoritarian personality will probably no longer fit in an organization that is evolving from a vertical, command/control structure to an information-based, fast-acting one. If the CFO pays lip service to independence and teamwork but still sends combative memos to staff in member hospitals, he is dysfunctional in the new structure. No amount of counseling, education, or discussion will reduce the impact that his past training, personal values, and history have on his behavior. He must be replaced.

In other cases, managers' technical skills might be excellent, but their values cause them to be dysfunctional and disruptive. A hard-nosed MBA with a for-profit bent may seem to be everything you want in a new business director, but her experiences may run counter to the organization's culture of shared responsibility. As a result, she may well become frustrated with the organization, making demands that are impossible to fulfill.

Like everything else, people, jobs, and organizations change. The environment exerts unending and irregular pressures on organizations. In response, organizations must redesign their cultures and "retool" to sustain followership. New cultures and structures call for new kinds of behaviors. Today's healthcare leaders must figure out what the organization needs and help people change to meet the future. In the same way, leaders must evaluate workers on two criteria: (1) what they are now and (2) what they must become if they are to contribute to the organization in the years ahead. Jack Welch (1996), past chairman of General Electric, says that there are four types of employees and describes them as follows:

1. High performers who share the company's values
2. High performers who do not share the values

3. Low performers who share the values
4. Low performers who do not share the values

Welch says numbers 1 and 4 are easy to deal with—promote number 1 and fire number 4. He recommends finding a place for number 3—finding people who share the company's values is too difficult not to keep the ones you have. Welch says that the hardest person to deal with is the high performer who does not share the values; in the case of healthcare, this could describe a physician. He suggests that each case be handled individually.

Finally, leaders must think about what their organization will become and communicate this vision in all things—especially in the use of human capital. A leader knows that because healthcare is a service business, the corporation's greatest assets are not on the balance sheet; they are walking the halls. Healthcare leaders are rethinking who they are, what business they are in, and whether they have the right team. Once they have defined their business and culture, they must clarify the roles of each team member and inspire followers to execute these roles. Remember: leaders inspire followers.

One of the leader's most elemental tasks is to balance what the organization expects of its employees with the employees' capacity to meet those expectations. Followers thrive when their values are matched carefully to a job. These followers will rarely quit or become troublemakers because they feel committed and bonded to the organization. If an organization has a reputation as a "revolving door," its titled executives must question their leadership ability. What happens between the time new employees walk into their office and the day they return their ID badges to security? The events between these two points define the executive's ability to lead.

Unfortunately, in approaching recruitment, the titled healthcare executive uses the warm-body approach: If the applicants are breathing and have the right credentials, they are hired. However, there is a step that must be taken before employees are hired:

Formulate the organization's purpose (values and mission) and set its direction (vision). *Then,* the best and the brightest people are found to achieve the vision. Trustees sometimes hire heavy-hitter CEOs from larger, more prosperous institutions only to fire them for bringing the organization "too far too fast" and for "stepping on toes." In the same way, senior executives bring in super-stars with skills and talent but no sense of team play.

Leaders explore how the concepts of person, job, and organization apply to their own situation. In doing so, they resist such hasty conclusions as "we need 25 new nurses" or "we've got to get a marketing vice president with a manufacturing background."

When addressing human resources and other issues, leaders ask the following questions:

- Is it a person, a job, or the organization that needs changing?
- What should the organization become?
- Do existing jobs match our mission, values, and vision?
- Do we have the right people to perform these jobs? If not, can these individuals be trained or coached, or should they be dismissed compassionately and replaced with others who fit the organization better?

Job Satisfaction and Commitment

Job satisfaction is the intangible result of a strong match between the person, the job, and the organization; it measures how happy employees are with their jobs, pay, coworkers, and supervisors. Commitment is a measure of employee loyalty, pride, and ownership. Staff will be satisfied and committed when their jobs provide them with the opportunity to be self-managed and empower them to achieve the organization's vision. To the surprise of many executives, there is a unique dynamic between commitment and job satisfaction. When taken together, staff who are neither loyal nor satisfied need to be paid more just to do the job.

Executives spend thousands of dollars on compensation studies when they should focus on the match between an employee's expectations and a job's opportunities. For example, if a nurse's personal need to care for patients matches the experiences available from working in an oncology unit, she will enjoy high job satisfaction, take pride in her work, and accept reasonable pay rates. But if she is rotated through various units with no attention to how her needs match those of the unit, she will probably feel used and demand a pay differential. The message is clear: Followers result from feeling needed, respected, and developed. If the inherent aspects of the job do not provide these elements, the tangible paycheck must compensate for the few intangibles, or people will leave.

People, then, work for both *financial* income and *psychic* income. Psychic income results from the combination of commitment and job satisfaction. The less psychic income that employees receive, the more financial income they will demand. Leaders are generous with both but emphasize psychic income.

Even in the executive ranks, psychic rewards are highly important. When a senior executive feels anxious about her work, she will continue to seek greater compensation or perks inside the organization, or she will look outside for a more lucrative opportunity. The absence of intrinsic rewards coupled with chronic anxiety about performance will cause her to demand higher and higher pay. Bolster and Hawthorne (2002) find that "Pay's up, satisfaction's down: From a compensation point of view, 2002 was a very good year for healthcare. But does it feel that way? Boards are uncomfortable, executives and managers continue to believe they deserve more, and increased pay hasn't reduced the growing dissatisfaction in the workforce. If the 8.1 percent base salary hike they got last year wasn't enough, what will be? Or must we reframe the debate from a market-competitive pay strategy to the role of reward in creating a compelling workplace?" Herein lies both the problem and the solution: Increasing satisfaction requires less focus on the tangibles and more focus on the intangibles.

Effective leaders are defined more by the commitment they engender in their followers than by the satisfaction they derive from their jobs. A director of dietary services may be satisfied with his job but feel no commitment to the organization. He would have few reservations about going to a competitor to perform the same duties for a relatively modest increase in pay or for some other reward. Many "climate" surveys of hospitals with high turnover rates leave executives baffled because employees report that they are satisfied with their jobs. What these surveys fail to ask is a critical follow-up question: Are you committed to the success of this organization? Commitment is the number one byproduct of effective leadership, and it is characterized by loyalty and pride.

Job satisfaction is typically measured by questions such as the following:

- Is there a match between your skills and experience?
- What does this job give you an opportunity to do?
- Do you like your boss?
- Is your compensation fair?
- Do you have a friend at work?

Organizational commitment, in contrast, is measured by questions such as the following:

- What would cause you to leave this organization?
- Do you understand this organization's purpose and beliefs?
- Are you proud of this organization?

Employee groups that exhibit high levels of satisfaction but low levels of commitment place the organization at risk. People in these groups tend to retreat into small enclaves for support. They reinforce one another with comments such as, "Just do your job"; "We don't know what they're doing over there, but we know our job"; "Let's just do our work and go home"; or "A day's work for a day's pay."

Mind Stretcher

Consider your own level of job satisfaction and organizational commitment by responding yes or no to the following statements taken from MetriTech's Healthcare Organizational Assessment Survey (Braskamp and Maehr 1986, 6–7):*

Job Satisfaction
- My coworkers and I work well together.
- I feel I get sufficient pay for the work I do.
- I like what I'm doing here, so I don't think of doing anything else.
- I get rewarded in a fair way for the work I do.
- I like my chances of doing work here so I can get ahead.
- I'm satisfied with the opportunities I have to direct people in my work.
- I get along with my supervisor.
- I like the people I work with.
- I like the work I do.
- I have good job security.

Organizational Commitment
- I have a sense of loyalty to this organization.
- I identify with this organization.
- I think about the future of this organization.
- I regret that I chose to work with this organization.
- I like to work here because I want the organization to succeed.
- I feel that I share in the success and failure of this organization.
- I feel that I have a sense of ownership in this organization.
- It would take a great deal for me to move to another organization.
- I take pride in being part of this organization.

---

* Copyright © 1985 MetriTech, Inc., Champaign, IL. Reproduced by permission.

Employees may like their job and coworkers but still feel no sense of identification with or loyalty to the organization. Those in the executive ranks may be in a slightly different situation. Traumatized by relentless change, they become obsessed with the details of their job and ignore the broader purposes of the organization. Continually looking ahead to the next meeting, financial statement, board agenda, or medical staff report, they manage their way through 12-hour days. Because they have no idea of how their job fits the organization's purpose, their only recourse is to work harder, longer, and faster and become even busier. Such managers approach their job like a student cramming for finals: I just need to get a passing grade and move on. No commitment, no passion, no leadership.

When people leave an organization or begin to look for a new job, it is usually because they experience low psychic income and the financial income is not high enough to justify working in a toxic environment. People do not leave organizations; they leave their boss, and this is clearly a reflection of low psychic income. The comments that follow, made to friends and colleagues during exit interviews, are telling:

> "Integrity is the first and critical factor in creating followers. This is why the first impression you make to a group is so important. They must see you as honest and competent. And I believe a seldom mentioned but very important factor is the leader must be humble."
>
> —*Jeffrey K. Norman, executive vice president, St. Vincent's Health System, Jacksonville, Florida*

Growth: "There's no opportunity for me to advance here. I'm going to look for another job."
Satisfaction: "If I stay here, they're going to have to pay me more, because I'm not happy with my job and I want more money."
Productivity: "I'm not productive here. I'm going to look for a job that values my contributions."
Frustration: "There's no relief in sight. Things aren't going to get better."

Priorities: "The organization needs skills I don't have, and I don't want to take the time, energy, and dollars to develop those skills."

Philosophy: "I don't like the way healthcare is going: I don't want to be part of it. I just want out."

Executives with few leadership skills will probably answer the following questions in quite different ways from inspirational leaders:

- What are my beliefs and values?
- What can I achieve as an executive, and where can I do it?
- What am I really worth—as a person and as a professional?
- What are my most significant skills and talents?
- Does this job give me the opportunity to use my strengths on the job at least 80 percent of the time?

Although some executives continually seek new opportunities, others will try to mold an organization to fit their personality and values. It is not uncommon to hear about the bright, aggressive, highly verbal CEO who runs a small community hospital as an entrepreneurial machine. Instead of leaving to become a superstar in a large organization, this leader makes the organization so vigorous and forward looking that he is never bored. He creates the conditions (defines the culture and builds the team) that make him more satisfied and committed.

Without commitment, an organization has nothing. High satisfaction without commitment will produce little more than a group of people who, when satisfiers weaken, may walk away and never take the time to wave goodbye. When staff are committed to an organization, however, there is unlimited potential for growth. The truly valuable manager is one who can say, "I believe in this place. The only way I would leave here is if the leadership changed." She may not be completely satisfied with her job, but she knows in which direction things are headed. She will invest her time, talent, and energy to help create a more effective organization because her deep belief in the leader's vision takes priority over superficial, tangible satisfiers.

Job satisfaction and commitment measures can also be used to anticipate and predict behavior. If employees have low organizational commitment, they may be candidates for union-organizing activities. If employees have high job satisfaction and low commitment, the probability of union activity is especially strong because employees will want to protect their job. People with high commitment may not be satisfied with their job, but they love the organization and will put in time to make it more effective. Those with high satisfaction and low commitment are more likely to complain, "Why are we having all of these meetings? I have work to do. I need to pay attention to my job, so stop bugging me with this mission stuff; it has nothing to do with me."

> "Mission, Values, Vision and Strength of Culture are our organizational centerpiece. Before a decision is made, it must pass the test that it strengthens our culture as defined by the mission, values and vision. If a decision runs counter to these factors or weakens them, it is not made."
>
> —*Kelly Mather, CEO, Sutter Lakeside Hospital, Lakeport, California*

To build a more effective organization, a leader needs to produce both high job satisfaction and high commitment. Keeping workers happy by itself is not the answer, and, in many cases, the existence of such workers may actually indicate an unwillingness to go the distance for the organization. If an executive is satisfied with his job but lacks commitment to the organization, he will eventually move elsewhere. Or if a titled executive, without a solid values-based mission and supporting vision remains with an organization, he could someday be among the corps of shell-shocked executives who cry out, "How can you treat me like this? I've given my life to this organization. Doesn't that mean anything?"

Strengthening Your Culture

What makes a strong culture? Service awards? Holiday parties? Monthly staff and management meetings? A calendar of staff birthdays displayed in the coffee room? Unfortunately, none of these things—alone or in combination—will create a strong culture. A salad bar in the cafeteria, a better parking spot, and an office with a view are the visual artifacts of an organization's climate—the things that can be seen. A culture, however, is based on beliefs. A strong culture exists when the following conditions are present:

- The organization has a clear sense of direction.
- Followers have clear expectations.
- Followers' behavior displays the values in everything they do.

If a strong culture exists, followers will answer yes to the following three questions:

1. Do I understand the mission, values, and vision of this organization?
2. Do I share these values?
3. Do I demonstrate them in my behavior?

In recent years, the cultures of healthcare organizations have been under almost continual attack. Titled executives thought they understood what hospitals did and why they existed. But what happens when the 200-bed hospital that stood at the corner of Main Street for 80 years is forced to close, and the other hospital in town finds it necessary to open a clinic in the mall? Titled executives in their late 40s and 50s have been known to say, "I don't know what hospitals are anymore. I spend several years of my life getting an education and more than 20 years in management, and I don't know where we're going or what we believe in."

Given their confusion about healthcare, hospitals, and their professional roles, it is no wonder that these titled executives find it difficult to build a strong culture where everyone shares the same values. The problem is that culture development must start at the top—not in human resources and not with a one-size-fits-all service management improvement program. A leader's most critical role is to define the culture, communicate the culture, and reward the followers who move the organization forward in the context of that culture. *A strong culture can never develop unless a leader first envisions it, articulates it, and lives it.*

What happens if the CEO abrogates this responsibility? Most likely, a mosaic of subcultures will emerge. No one can live outside a values context, which means that no one can live without a belief system. If the CEO fails to define and promote a clear corporate culture, employees will often create conflicting subcultures. Confused by upper management's talk about "a decentralized, polycorporate environment," finance may create a subculture devoted to controlling debt and watching over the cash flow, budget, and accounts receivable. Other professionals and disciplines that are in the process of developing new identities, such as nursing, pharmacy, and physical therapy, will also create subcultures to define their context—the belief system that underpins their behavior.

An efficient organization can and should have many diverse personalities but only one corporate culture. In a strong culture, you can put people who are in clinical areas, support, or fund development in the same room, and they will continue to talk care, support, and fund development—but in the context of the organization's mission, values, and vision. In ineffective organizations, diverse subcultures are less benign. If the vision is to create a responsive, information-based organization and the CFO exercises neurotic control over cash, debt, and capital, problems will arise. If a titled executive wants to build a diversified business group to cover losses in acute care units and the medical staff resists, there will be other kinds of problems. Dynamic tension is healthy for an organization as long as the members respond, in unison, How does this help our purpose? Is this what we're working for? When subcultures clash, the organization weakens.

In describing strong cultures, people often speak of vitality, exuberance, soul, energy, heart, magic, and life. In short, strong cultures have *spirit*. They are very busy and possess a dynamic energy, even though their employees are relaxed, open, and friendly. Employees understand the big picture and do everything they can to help each other and the people they serve. Successful teams are not those with the greatest skill but those with the best spirit. If one team has 100 players who are confused, apathetic, and unfocused and the other team has 10 players who display a "magical" quality about winning, which team has the better odds of thriving? It is never size—it is always spirit.

> "Leaders think of the team first. They listen and understand individual needs as they relate to team success. They set direction and hold people accountable while constantly supporting and developing the team members' potential."
>
> —Julianna Castro, APN, nurse practitioner, Genesis Health Group, Silvis, Illinois

The hallmark of an effective organization is a focused, satisfied, and committed workforce that follows a courageous, energetic, and disciplined leader. If employees, physicians, and trustees are satisfied and committed, they will not only be productive but will thrive on change. Unfortunately, many titled executives introduce change with no understanding of corporate values and what motivates employees. When resistance mounts, they wail, "My staff is organizing. They don't understand. Why are they fighting me on this? I just spent $100,000 on a strategic plan and they won't implement it." If an executive pushes through a plan and ignores issues of values, satisfaction, commitment, and culture, he will likely double or triple the plan's original costs in turnover, reduced productivity, and internal strife and still never be able to implement the plan. Leaders realize that it is easy to formulate ideas and plans, but success is found in implementation through followers.

CEOs who are hired into healthcare organizations with unfamiliar cultures have two choices: Adapt to the current culture and put a distinctive trademark on it or create a new culture. Some CEOs make the transition, but others crash and burn within months, usually over a culture-related, values-based issue. The CEO who was once viewed by the board as the hope for the future quickly becomes the maniac who went out of control. The aggressive, entrepreneurial problem solver who was hired to catapult the organization into the twenty-first century is berated for "moving us too far too fast." CEOs are much more likely to lose their job because of a "personality conflict" than lack of competence. Ninety percent of hiring decisions are based on the tangibles (credentials, experience), and 90 percent of termination decisions are based on the intangibles (values clash and communication style).

CONCLUSION

Since behavior is driven by values, leaders should take time out once a year to do a total assessment of person, job, and organization to see how the values function and fit. They must be willing to ask some hard questions: How strong is the organization's culture? Do various subcultures have a negative impact? Are employees divisive, or are they willing to support the organization's mission? Where are values strong, and where are they weak? Can the mission be achieved? Are the *right people* in the *right job* doing the *right things*? Does the organization have a soul? If yes, is it headed for heaven or hell?

REFERENCES

Bolster, C. J., and G. Hawthorne. 2002. "2002 Executive Compensation Survey. Can Money Buy Happiness?" *Trustee* 55 (10): 8–12.

Braskamp, L.A., and M. L. Maehr. 1986. The Healthcare Organizational Assessment Survey. Champaign, IL: MetriTech, Inc.

Welch, J. 1996. "General Electric Corporate Annual Report." February. General Electric Company.

PART TWO

Measuring Followership

CHAPTER 5

Measuring the Intangibles: Creating Sustainable Change

SUCCESSFUL HEALTHCARE LEADERS are defined by their ability to create a corporate culture in which followership thrives. The previous chapters focus on the characteristics and behaviors that result in a "follower-rich ecosystem." Theoretical and field research shows that trust in the leader is the most critical element that differentiates healthcare leaders (i.e., those with followers) and titled executives (i.e., those with position but few followers). Closely behind trust as success factors are integrity, consistency, ethical behavior, and humility. Leaders who exhibit these traits are more successful at creating a followership than those who engender fear, uncertainty, and doubt in their employees. These intangibles underpin sustainable corporate success and make sustainable change possible.

Valid, periodic measures of these intangible factors are necessary to determine the strength of the corporate culture and the degree that the current culture is supporting a positive (i.e., follower friendly) work environment. Recall from Figure 1.1 the major tangible, intangible, and corporate soul elements of a work environment. The major premise of Part II of this book focuses on measuring and managing the intangible and corporate soul elements, which must be handled with the same diligence that is used with the tangibles. The old mantra of "no margin, no mission" justifies obsessive measurement and analysis of the tangibles (especially finances). The new mantra, "no balance, no business," demands that the tangibles, intangibles, and corporate soul be measured with the same enthusiasm and rigor.

MEASURING THE INTANGIBLES

Figure 5.1 shows that corporate soul and intangible elements are the nonfinancial reasons for work. They define the reasons that leaders have followers. This figure shows just the inputs and outputs for the corporate soul and the intangibles. Can you identify a metric or measurement methodology used in your organization for each of the elements listed? How many of these elements are measured and reported quarterly to the board? The easiest way to do a quick analysis of the corporate culture of any healthcare organization is to observe two variables: (1) what data are taken to the board, shared with the staff, and presented to the community and (2) what achievements are celebrated. It is my belief that you are what you measure and you are what you celebrate. Very simply, the understanding of the relationship between a strong corporate culture and followership requires measurement and analysis of the intangible and corporate soul factors and celebration of improvement in the intangible and corporate soul elements.

Consider Greg Carlson, CHE, president and CEO of Owensboro Mercy Health System (OMHS) in Owensboro, Kentucky. He has created an almost perfect balance between the tangible and intangible elements of his organization. If you followed him around for a while, you would learn that his passion for productivity and accountability is framed by an optimistic belief in the potential of people. He understands very clearly that effective organizations must take into account all of the elements listed in Figure 5.1. Carlson is a leader; Carlson has many followers.

Figure 5.1: Two of the Three Work Environment Domains

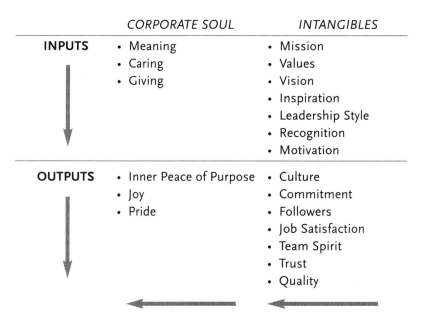

	CORPORATE SOUL	*INTANGIBLES*
INPUTS	• Meaning • Caring • Giving	• Mission • Values • Vision • Inspiration • Leadership Style • Recognition • Motivation
OUTPUTS	• Inner Peace of Purpose • Joy • Pride	• Culture • Commitment • Followers • Job Satisfaction • Team Spirit • Trust • Quality

Source: Adapted from Atchison, T. 2001. "Striking a Balance." *Trustee* 54 (7): 28. Reprinted from *Trustee*, Vol. 54 No. 7, by permission, July/August 2001, Copyright 2001, by Health Forum, Inc.

Leaders have followers who make a strong commitment to the organization. When this occurs, the organization has a strong culture, and employees will exhibit job satisfaction, pride, and high morale. Therefore, if a leader creates a strong culture, he will have followers—highly committed people who are proud to work for him and the organization.

A leader's employees will display the sense of respect, trust, and well-being that results from the unique form of energy created by team spirit. They believe in their leader and, without saying so directly, they acknowledge his ability to inspire the organization. Data from OMHS (Figure 5.2) show the growth of a corporate culture from the time Carlson became the senior executive and "chief leadership officer" responsible for followership.

Figure 5.2: OMHS's **Corporate Culture**

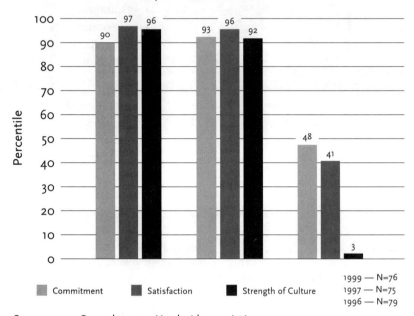

Owensboro Mercy Health System
Owensboro, KY

Total Group
Key Motivational Scales

Source: OMHS, Owensboro, KY. Used with permission.

OMHS created a corporate culture (i.e., work environment) that inspired followers, which increased pride and job satisfaction. One of the most misunderstood dynamics of leadership is the relationship between a strong corporate culture and financial viability. Leaders who focus on followership and creating a positive work environment are able to show larger-than-expected financial gains, whereas titled executives who focus on financial performance at the expense of the workforce show lower-than-expected financial gains. The intangibles always underpin sustainable business improvement. The OMHS data in Table 5.1 clearly demonstrate this dynamic.

Table 5.1: OMHS Financial Performance Data

	5/31/96	5/31/97	5/31/98*
Gross revenue	229.9	231.8	246,044
Net revenue	143.4	142.2	150,988
Profit	13.5	16.7	23.24
Profit as in % of net revenue	9.4	11.7	15.89
Number of executives	13	7	8
Number of FTEs (premerger = 1,935)	1,710	1,738	1,795**
Length of stay	4.6	4.3	4.1

Note: Revenue numbers are in millions.
* Projected based on six months' annualization
** Increase due to volume and new services such as urgent care, community wellness, sleep lab, inpatient chemical dependency, and other new or expanded services
Source: OMHS, Owensboro, KY. Used with permission.

From November 5, 1999, to September 2002, the following events took place that highlight accomplishments by OMHS:

- OMHS has reduced rates four times, reduced charges by $141.2 million, and reduced operating costs by $75.6 million, as determined by KPMG, a national auditing firm.
- OMHS has increased community benefit contributions from $700,000 per year prior to merger to $3 million for 2002.
- Charity care has virtually doubled since the merger to over $9 million in 2002.
- Compared to national standards, OMHS's average cost per case of $4,071 is nearly $1,000 lower than the national figure.
- OMHS has decreased length of stay from 4.8 days to 3.9 days.
- OMHS consistently maintains an employee turnover rate of 12 percent, which is lower than the Kentucky state average of 22 percent.

- Forty-five new physicians have joined OMHS's medical staff since the merger.
- OMHS has passed its last eight state licensure surveys (for home care, Official Medicines Control Laboratory, transitional care center, dialysis, radiation therapy, outpatient therapy, speech and audiology, and "convenient care") with no deficiencies.
- The Joint Commission on Accreditation of Healthcare Organizations awarded OMHS, its lab, and its home care full accreditation during its last survey.
- OMHS has received no audit adjustments from the accounting firm of KPMG Peat Marwick, LLP, on the past six financial audits.
- OMHS has been recognized for leadership in community service and given community health awardsby the Kentucky Hospital Association and the Voluntary Hospitals of America.
- Capital investments have been made to bring the latest healthcare technology to the community.
- Many new services, such as the sleep lab, the HealthPark, and the chemical dependency unit, have been added to better serve the community.

> "Leaders create followers because they first listen—not just hear, but truly listen. They then assimilate the many points of view and place the results in the context of the organization's vision. Finally, they are able to communicate the direction in ways that everyone understands the benefits."
>
> —Jack Kolosky, executive vice president of planning and finance, H. Lee Moffitt Cancer Center and Research Institute, Tampa, Florida

To achieve these intangible and tangible gains, Carlson turns to his followers often and asks the following questions:

- Do we share the organization's beliefs?
- Do we display our values in everything we do?
- Do we like working here?

- Are we proud of our work?
- Are we happy about working here?
- Is trust prevalent throughout the organization?

If you ask these questions and most of the workforce answers yes, they are followers who have committed themselves to the vision of the organization. The conclusion would be different if the workforce answers the questions with, "I don't know and I don't care."

Unfortunately, many healthcare organizations do not measure their success on the basis of intangible factors such as culture, job satisfaction, and commitment. Instead, they measure success on the basis of financially oriented, tangible variables such as profit, increased market share, and productivity.

The reality is that an organization may perform successfully in many of these areas but still lack leadership. An even deeper reality is that organizations that lose control of, minimize, or ignore the intangible factors will, over time, suffer in the tangible output sector. If the culture is weak and people feel no pride in their work and no commitment to the organization, market share, profit, and productivity are at great risk. The situation is like a snake eating its own tail: It believes it is satisfying its appetite, until it bites its head.

ACHIEVING EFFECTIVENESS

The process for creating a more effective organization involves three phases—assessment, analysis, and action. Each phase will be introduced in the following sections and discussed more fully in chapters 6, 7, and 8. It begins with a thorough examination of the intangible elements that characterize such an organization. In medicine, treatment without diagnosis is malpractice. The same principle holds true for healthcare organizations. Unless data are first gathered about the intangibles of the organization, a diagnosis and a practical course of treatment can never be developed. Just as a physician examines and talks with the patient, so a leader must scrutinize and interact with every component of the organization.

Central to this process are several issues: What is really happening to this organization? How are people being affected by the increasing pressure in healthcare to do more with less? Most importantly, what is my leader's personal style of leadership? Is it helping or hindering the organization in achieving its mission, fulfilling its values, and moving toward its vision?

ASSESSMENT: DEFINE YOUR TARGET

Although the word *assessment* may awaken painful memories of third-grade multiplication test or grades hidden from parents, organizational assessment is a direct, benign, and clear-cut process. Reduced to its simplest terms, organizational assessment involves two steps: (1) the intangibles that underpin the organization's behavior must first be translated into numbers and (2) it must be established which of the numbers are most meaningful to the organization's vision.

Essential to the assessment process is a leader's candid look at her own leadership style. In performing this self-appraisal, she must confront such basic issues as how she expresses her feelings and beliefs, communicates the vision, recognizes and rewards high performers, disciplines with compassion, and celebrates team accomplishments. Caution is necessary here. In digging beneath the surface, leaders may uncover troubling truths about how they are perceived by others. They should consider the following questions:

- Do people in the organization really take pride in their work?
- What is my role in facilitating pride in the workplace?
- To what extent do I meet the varying perceptions and expectations of the professional, management, technical,

clerical, and support staff? How do these perceptions and expectations shape the behavior of the workforce?

- How do I typically refer to workers in conversations with colleagues, senior management, physicians, and trustees? What do these labels indicate about my attitudes, beliefs, and values?

- Do I view workers (and physicians) simply as necessary evils or as cogs in the organizational machine? If not, how is their status as partners (especially physicians) in fulfilling the organization's mission reinforced?

- How much credit is the workforce given for organizational excellence? Am I fulfilling the leader's role as orchestra conductor? How much acknowledgment do the musicians get as the primary reason for the organization's success?

- What specific actions have been taken in the last week, the last month, and the last year to show workers and physicians that they are valued? What have been the results of these efforts?

Assessing an organization involves measuring its intangible aspects (see Figure 5.1). Assessment is the process whereby behaviors are converted into measurable, quantifiable statements. These raw data become the basis for analysis, judgment, and action plans. The difficult aspects of assessment are ensuring that whatever you decide to measure is in fact what you are measuring, that the results are valid and reliable for your organization, and that the data allow you to compare your organization to some accepted norm. These conditions must exist before informed interpretations of the data can be made.

Shooting from the Hip

Titled executives sometimes approach organizational assessment as though it were a gunfight at high noon. Instead of using valid data addressing the factors that can result in victory or defeat, they come out with guns blazing and, in classic shoot-from-the-hip style, look for the most convenient or obvious target—for example, "nurse morale is bad!" As a result, many titled healthcare executives never take their finger off the trigger long enough to understand their organization's most troublesome intangible weaknesses or its deepest reservoirs of intangible strengths. Such lack of focus costs time, money, and effort. Recall the medical model. Treatment without diagnosis is malpractice. In the same way, in the executive ranks, data about the intangibles, converted by analysis into information, must drive every change program. If you do not measure, you cannot manage. Without data, titled executives default to subjective impressions.

One Size Fits All

Someday we may live in a world where organizational development programs will be like pantyhose and stretch underwear: One size fits all. Unfortunately, like the less-than-perfect individuals who try to fit themselves into these miracles of Seventh Avenue marketing efforts, healthcare employees often feel squashed and uncomfortable when forced to undertake generic change programs. To address a complex intangible problem with a one-size-fits-all tangible solution is *always* a waste of time and money.

The matter of customer service provides an example. Convinced that Marriott, Disneyland, and some hospital programs held the magic elixir to cure healthcare's ills, self-styled customer service experts proceeded to wrap every wounded hospital with the same bandage. All too often, employees reacted with anger and resentment: "My mother taught me how to smile," "I don't need a script to do my job," "This isn't a hotel," and "We're not in Florida!" The only truly effective patient satisfaction programs are those that are designed, pilot tested, and evaluated by the healthcare professionals who will use them. In these cases, the employees pinpointed the real problems, generated support from the lowest levels of the organization, and then concluded, "We need a tiny refinement in this area and a major overhaul here." They owned the program—they were committed. All the leader did was to use the core values to inspire them to think about improving service.

This is not to say that there is no value in prefabricated programs. Workbooks—now frequently backed by computer software—can be helpful if managers use them to generate basic awareness, create insights, or remedy general problems. There is no reason to develop a completely new program if one with a good track record of success already exists. But permanent change only happens when the work is tailored to an organization's culture. Successful change comes from commitment, and commitment comes from ownership.

Smoking causes almost 400,000 deaths a year, and morbid obesity is a risk factor for stroke, heart attacks, and diabetes. Does this mean that everyone who tries to quit smoking or lose weight should go through hypnosis, biofeedback, acupuncture, massage therapy, or any number of other programs popular at the moment? The answer is no. Different techniques and strategies work for different people. The upwardly mobile young accountant who successfully lost weight by means of a modified fast and liquid protein supplements may have a personality, an education, and a socioeconomic background that contributed to his success. The same program might not work for a hospital cafeteria worker whose identity revolves around cooking glorious meals for his family.

"Followers result from being honest and forthright. This is especially true for physicians. They must trust you to follow you. It takes a lot of energy to get a core of physicians to support the corporate strategic plan. It all starts with honesty, which includes an understanding that we agree to disagree without getting personal."

—*Scott Nygaard, M.D., chief medical officer and senior vice president of medical affairs, Affinity Health System, Menasha, Wisconsin*

The analogy also applies to organizations. The 325-bed hospital in an upscale suburb wins over its employees with a sophisticated health promotion program that includes personal diaries, progress logs, and regular visits to a local health club. In a bungalowed suburb where employees come from old-fashioned Eastern European families, the same program falls flat. Why the different results? Because of the different preferences, values, and backgrounds of the employees, and also because of the different missions, values, and visions of the organizations and the kinds of people they tend to attract and retain.

The healthcare industry displays an intriguing paradox. Self-righteous titled executives are admonished to review an organization's financial statements for days just to leverage an additional two points off an investment. Yet when it comes to human capital, motivation, pride, commitment, and a host of other intangible factors, that same organization treats all its employees alike. "We have a morale problem here" is how titled CEOs typically articulate a broad array of undifferentiated, intangible concerns. But not everyone in the organization may suffer from a morale problem; furthermore, not everyone should be prodded to adopt the same solution.

Currently, the most popular form of generic change programs turns on compensation. Now viewed as the panacea for the nursing crisis, the idea that money buys happiness will soon find its way into recruitment and retention programs for medical technologists, family practitioners, pharmacists, and respiratory therapists. Unfortunately, this approach is an extension of a larger societal concept that views money as a one-way ticket to a better life. As experience demonstrates, however, throwing money at a personnel problem never solves it. Intangible problems such as lack of commitment cannot be solved by tangible inputs such as cash. In almost all cases, executives must instead attack the larger issues of organizational structure and make sure that people fit into a values context that promotes commitment and increases self-esteem.

One hospital CEO thought that he had solved his nurse retention problem by giving his nurses handsome raises. At one time, the hospital made money with a 65 percent occupancy rate, but now it needs more than 80 percent occupancy to meet its profitability goals. What will happen when the nurses' morale needs another boost and the hospital needs a 105 percent occupancy rate to turn a profit? You need not be an accountant to figure out that this CEO is caught in a powerful undertow. The message is simple: If you throw money at an intangible problem now, you will probably end up throwing more money at that same problem in the future. Employees may come to expect not only a decent wage but regular, generous increases as well. Satisfaction can be bought in the short term, but long-term commitment must be earned.

ANALYSIS

Analysis requires both evaluation and judgment. Consider this example: Following an annual physical, a physician tells the patient that his cholesterol level is 340. The number is nothing more than the quantification of a condition at that moment in time. It is when the physician says, "You know, this is quite serious." This is an evaluation, a judgment. The physician is explaining that the number represents a negative or harmful situation. In assessment, behavior is frozen in time and then quantified. In the analysis phase, the raw data are evaluated and a determination is made whether the data signify that the behavior is acceptable. Analysis is needed to interpret what those numbers mean in terms of the corporate culture. It is during the analysis phase that the following questions are asked and answered:

> "Followers work hard in a workplace because they have a deep commitment to the organizational mission and vision, and they embrace the organization's values. Or, desperate people can work hard because they're afraid of being fired. Where would you rather work?"
>
> —Robert Bonar, PH.D., president and CEO, Children's Hospital of Austin, Texas

1. Why does our organization exist? (mission)
2. What do we believe in? (values)

3. Where are we headed? (vision)
4. Does everyone answer these questions in the same way? (strength of culture)

These are the four toughest questions that leaders must ask.

If some titled healthcare executives try to fit every organizational recruit into the same bland uniform, others tiptoe on the surface of problems like mice on cotton. What they fail to take into account is that most organizations exist on three levels: (1) the artifacts or "climate" level that is apparent to everyone, (2) the values level that drives behavior, and (3) the deep structure created by a mosaic of independent personalities. Why do some executives never delve below the first level? In most cases, it is easier to grapple with the more superficial issues related to job satisfaction. The question, What would it take to make you happy? usually elicits familiar answers: a child-care center, better food in the cafeteria, a more convenient parking place, or more pay. While these are important, they have less to do with building commitment than with job satisfaction. Commitment comes from engendering feelings of respect and providing chances to grow as a professional.

In contrast, consider the responses provoked by these questions: What would increase your pride, loyalty, and commitment to this organization? What would it take to really "turn you on" to work? Few employees would mention the quality of the coffee, summertime baseball outings, or Christmas bonuses. Instead, if questioned in depth, they might talk about their desire to share tasks with other professionals and enrich their work life by learning new skills. Of course, none of these are easy solutions. You will not find them in the latest management best seller about increasing productivity because they come from the heart and soul of your employees. The problem is that soliciting employees' ideas takes time. Putting their ideas into practice takes even longer.

Is it any wonder, therefore, that titled executives take the easy and most obvious way out? But if their analytical approach finds solutions only at the simplest level, they will get snared in a never-ending struggle to make people happy. Failure is inevitable because, as noted before, employees' expectations begin to escalate. Because they are neither self-managed nor self-motivated, these individuals continually look to various kinds of external satisfiers for compensation. A worker motivation plan based almost entirely on external rewards will limit staff behavior. So what choice do staff members have but to ask for more and more?

In contrast, a strong, values-based culture defines the context for appropriate behavior. In a values-based culture, people focus on how their work contributes to the organization and how the organization improves personal feelings of worth. Remember that employees work to increase their psychic income. The more they are treated like doormats, the more they want to be paid, because their only feelings of worth come from their paychecks. Why do people attend a particular religious service? Because of the deeper dimensions of values alignment and pride. No one goes to a particular church because they pay the most for each hour of service attended.

The final question for executives in the course of analysis is this: Do we have the right people doing the right job at the right time? If you focus on the happiness quotient on the satisfiers, people may be happy but will not necessarily be committed to the organization. If you focus on matching core corporate values with employee values, however, staff will be both happy *and* committed.

Treating a troubled organization with special programs such as stress management seminars, employee service awards, and Christmas get-togethers at the president's house is like trying to treat cardiac disease exclusively with rest. The treatment has merit but is not sufficient. To recover completely, the heart patient needs a total life change brought about by changes in the way he eats, exercises, and manages stress. In the same way, the titled executive will never achieve success by investing in the management development "program of the month" and hiding behind the costly armor of new workbooks, videos, and overheads.

For leaders to change their organizations, they must be willing to take risks and be prepared for a long struggle. Leaders resist the temptation to delegate the task to a senior associate, vice president of human resources, or even their favorite administrative assistant. A leader's chief task is to discover what it is that will energize the organization. No focused effects will occur without leadership, but the results will be worth the effort. Remember, culture drives behavior, and culture begins and ends with leadership.

> "Organizational values need to be practiced at all levels of the organization. Most importantly, your actions must reinforce what you say—you are your behavior. Eliminate rules and bureaucracy—most rules send the message that you don't trust them. And never use one-size-fits-all programs with staff. Treat them as you would like to be treated, and they will follow you anywhere."
>
> —*Greg Carlson*, CHE, *president and* CEO, *Owensboro Mercy Health System, Owensboro, Kentucky*

ACTION

It is during the action phase that leaders develop and implement the program for change. They identify and analyze barriers to achieving the vision and list the essential change elements, which are the positive alternatives to behaviors that are blocking progress. Barriers are key bottlenecks that, when removed, have dramatic effects. Note however that some barriers cannot be removed or shifted. Federal regulations are one example—they must be accepted and coped with. These change elements form a bridge between the organization's present and its future. The intangibles of mission, values, and vision address four issues: Why do we exist? What do we believe in? Where are we headed? What are the barriers or obstacles that we must eliminate, reduce, or accept? Essential change elements complete the statement, "To move forward, we must start to do, continue to do, or, stop doing." Whether they involve hard assets or intangibles such as trust and cooperation, essential change elements redirect energy from barriers toward action.

Insight into the barriers to change and identification of the essential change elements create the road map for action. The next step, as the Nike commercial says, is to "Just do it."

Fixing Blame Versus Taking the High Road

When taking action, some executives find it easier to fix blame than fix the problem. After all, if a person can place the responsibility on someone else, he can remain innocent—at least for awhile. For example, if a titled executive can convince others that most of the problems at his hospital are the work of troublesome, greedy physicians and unreasonable regulations, he can then disclaim all responsibility for causing the problems or for finding solutions to them. Furthermore, he can minimize his own sense of failure or disappointment because the problem never had anything to do with him. After all, "It was those doctors. If they had the sense to stick to the business of practicing medicine," he tells board members, "this could have been avoided. We are victims—powerless!"

At one time or another, we have all played this game. We do it with such ease and innocence that it is often difficult to catch ourselves. Consider these examples: A student fails an exam because "the teacher didn't explain the material clearly." A woman remains overweight because "this situation is driving me crazy. I have to eat to forget it." An employee is continually tardy because "I have so much work that I am always tired and wake up late."

To rely on these excuses and pass blame on to others is very human, but executives who engage in this behavior on a regular basis are executives in title only. Why? Because they refuse to accept that they may be part of the problem. More importantly, they have abdicated their responsibility to create positive change.

One should ask oneself, Is it always someone else's problem? Do I tend to use phrases such as, "That's a decision *you'll* have to make for yourself"; "The problem with *those people* is that they won't change"; "*They* don't understand what we're doing over here"; "Why can't *they* get with the program?"; "We need people who can take this organization in the right direction"; and "I'm a good leader, but I wish I had better followers"?

If the problem is always with a person, department, organization, or entity that is supposedly outside the executive's control, something is seriously wrong. If replacing employees, restructuring the organization, or remodeling her office is the executive's treatment of choice, perhaps she needs to spend more time reflecting on her own behavior. Perhaps she should ask herself the following questions:

- When I accuse people of not wanting to change, have I really developed an adequate rationale for change?
- Do people feel secure and protected enough to make the change?
- Do they understand the direction and consequences of the change?
- If they don't understand the grand design for the organization, does this mean my communication style is inadequate?
- How can I determine which communication channels are inadequate?
- How can rumors and misperceptions be controlled and corrected?
- What steps can be taken to make people feel more invested and involved?

> "Followers believe in a dream. They believe that the leader will take them to a better place. Followers trust that the leader is skilled enough to get them to 'the mountain' and cares enough about them to make the journey to 'the mountain' beneficial to each of them."
>
> —*Lynn M. Schroth*, DR.P.H., CHE, *executive vice president, The Methodist Hospital, Houston, Texas*

Leaders take ownership of behavior. An important aspect of their behavior is the quality and character of their language. Titled executives often become the victims of language, drowning in the latest management lingo about "self-starters" who can "hit the deck running" or mired in flowery clichés about the organization being a "real family." Most often, however, they are obsessed with what was or what might have been and constantly lament, "We should have done this last year" or "I wish the government would stop taking advantage of us."

Leaders take a different tack. Instead of going on nostalgic journeys through decades past, they use language to assume more responsibility and take aggressive action. Rather than trying to fix blame or spending their time in a fantasy world of how good it used to be, effective leaders focus on what is happening here and now and seek out the meaning of events and situations. They are likely to say, "There's nothing we can do to change the past. Things aren't the way they used to be, and we're going to have to accept that. But what we can do is create a more effective organization, and I'm going to make sure that people here get all the support they need to do it."

Leaders calm the troubled waters of organizations by their willingness to climb to the highest point of the mountain and see if the sun is peeking from behind a cloud or if storm clouds are on the horizon. They know that as the environment changes, the options for action also change. These days, healthcare needs more leaders who offer a mountain-top perspective. Without it, titled executives will continue to narrowly analyze staff motivation as a compensation problem and ignore more basic issues. Consider the question, How are we going to deliver quality healthcare to patients if key staff are no longer committed? The answer must be, Change the organization and clarify the roles and increase the pride in followers. Without an elevated perspective, titled executives will continue to seek the quick fix—which only serves as a temporary opiate. Sustainable change lies in the way that leaders measure and manage the intangibles.

CHAPTER 6

Assessment:
Conducting an Inventory of the
Organization and Yourself

FOLLOWERS WANT AND need feedback that answers such questions as, Where are we headed, why, what's my role, and how are we doing so far? Answering these and other work-related questions continually encourages followership, and periodic assessments of meaningful data are a useful source for finding those answers. The assessment data must, of course, meet the accepted standards for validity (i.e., measuring what we say we want to measure) and reliability (i.e., if we measure these variables over and over again, we will get very similar responses). Leaders realize that the assessments that most benefit the organization are those for intangibles, such as employee pride and patient satisfaction. The measurement of these intangibles, as well as the others in Figure 1.1, need to be completed with the same diligence and rigor that we currently measure the tangibles, such as budget variation and market share.

The introduction of an organizationwide assessment process must be done in a way that encourages followership. Too often, any measurement of the intangibles is viewed as not very useful. Prior to the administration of an assessment, leaders should survey the organization's environment to determine the readiness of staff for an assessment. They should ask questions such as the following:

- How am I planning to use this assessment? Is it a carrot or a club? Am I secretly hoping to flush out troublemakers and punish the guilty? Or am I committed to using this assessment as the first step in building a more effective organization through meaningful engagement of followers?
- Does this assessment have a clear-cut context and purpose? Have I communicated this context and purpose to every key member in the organization?
- Have I already fixed in my mind the nature of this organization's problems? Or am I truly open to the results of this assessment? Am I prepared to deal with the data—no matter how negative or threatening they may be?
- Are my expectations for the assessment realistic, specific, and attainable?
- Have I carefully identified the recipients and users of the data? Are they committed to the process and to the outcome of the assessment? How will I involve them in selecting the instrument, analyzing the data, and communicating the results?
- Have I explored how the data from the assessment will be analyzed and communicated? What channels of communication will be most effective?
- Have I taken the time to deal candidly with people's fears and concerns? Have I provided adequate assurance that no one will get hurt in the process? Do people understand that the goal of the process is not to fix blame or build secret personnel files but to create a better organization?
- What assurances do I have that the data will be valid and reliable? Does the instrument have a good track record in the healthcare industry? Is it reliable? If we were repeatedly to administer the same instrument, would it produce the same results?

- In sum, am I fully prepared to answer these questions about the assessment: Why are we carrying out the assessment? What are we going to assess? How should we structure this assessment? What will we do with the data?

ON THE ROAD TO MEANINGFUL ASSESSMENT

As the assessment process begins, there are several things to keep in mind.

Avoid satisfaction surveys. Instruments that are little more than Dr. Feelgood "climate" or satisfaction surveys should be avoided. Worrying about job satisfaction—how happy people are—will do little to enhance the likelihood of sustainable followership. But focusing on commitment factors, such as pride, loyalty, self-management, and affiliation, increases the chance that employees will become followers. If commitment drives a follower's professional life, she is likely to respond to an alluring job offer with, "Thanks, but I'm really involved here. I believe in this place. They're going through some hard times, and I want to see this thing through."

Employee attitudes are important, but attitudes alone will never give a total picture of what staff need to follow the leader. Nor will highly quantitative productivity profiles necessarily lead the way to future success. The starting point of any assessment of the intangibles is in values—who one is and what one believes in. These are the convictions that drive behavior. A disservice is done if productivity is measured without looking at why people are productive or unproductive. No contribution is made if attitudes are measured without looking at the deeper dimensions (i.e., values and beliefs) that support them.

Assessment data cannot do it all. Diagnosis, by itself, does not solve the problem. Knowing you have a disease does not cure the disease. Insight must be followed by action. Executives often think that they can fix human behavior as easily as a glazier can fix a broken window. Unfortunately, this is almost never the case. Typically, it takes about twice the amount of time to fix a problem as it did to create it.

Behavior changes slowly, except in the case of trauma. Of course, pain, shock, and trauma can be created by using terror tactics, but such strategies will not be worth the effort in the long term because the followership is situational and not based on values alignment. Change that follows trauma usually carries a heavy price tag. Ultimately, people will regress, rebel, or even engage in sabotage.

The primary purpose of assessment is to determine how well people fit within the organization. Thus, if an employee, physician, or board member has a personal history that directly conflicts with the organization, resist the temptation to bring the two together and then try to work a miracle. Leaders have better ways to invest their time, talent, and energy. Remember what Collins (2001) recommends in *Good to Great: Why Some Companies Make the Leap . . . and Others Don't:* Select the right people first.

> "First of all a CEO must lead by example. Followers are created by being consistent in what you do and how you do it."
>
> —William Foley, FACHE, president and CEO, Provena Health, Mokena, Illinois

Know the organization's assessment history. The leader needs to be aware of the history and tradition of assessments in the organization. A CEO who wanted to retain control of every management decision outraged his employees when he announced an upcoming assessment of the organization. Insulted and threatened by the process, employees viewed the assessment exercise as an opportunity to settle some old scores with the boss. They used the assessment not only to communicate a negative message but also to take revenge for the irritating way in which he meddled in their affairs.

In assessing the organization, a leader should be aware of people's attitudes toward and experiences with assessment tools used in the past. Typically, most people wince at the word *assess-*

ment. Like the student who is unprepared for a test, the reluctant employee will do everything from lashing out at the boss to spreading rumors about how the results will be used. On an even more basic level, most people like to think of themselves as unique or special. How could anyone reduce who they are and what they do to a survey, they wonder. The reality, of course, is that most human behavior—especially in the workplace—is fairly predictable.

Tie the assessment to the mission, values, and vision of the organization. For what purpose does our organization exist (mission)? What do we believe in (values)? Where are we headed (vision)? These questions are the essence of each phase of the assessment, analysis, and action process. If an executive engages one of his managers by using casual weekly charts on the topic of motivation, the information garnered is no doubt rich in interesting data. However, one issue will remain: What is the context for these data? Specifically, what is their meaning, and how does this information and data relate to the organization's mission, values, and vision?

Focus on the deeper motivational values that drive behavior. If followers are encouraged to be open and candid about what they think of the organization, can their feelings toward their boss, work, and organization really make a difference? In developing any assessment, you must first answer one question: Am I measuring attitudes or am I measuring behavior? Despite the lip service paid to "the magic of language," words are cheap in our society. Attention should be focused on behavior. What people do defines who they are.

Assess the situation before taking action. Sixty pounds overweight and a smoker for more than 20 years, Myra continually cancelled appointments with her physician. Finally, she admitted, "If I don't hear him tell me what's wrong, I don't have to deal with it." At least in the short-term, Myra functions better by avoiding diagnosis and assessment of something she already understands on an intuitive level.

Many executives—especially those at the helm of dysfunctional organizations—are surprisingly like Myra. By avoiding a values-based assessment process, they postpone confrontation with the truth. At least for a short time, they can hold fast to the status quo. However, by refusing to do an assessment, the titled executive has abdicated his role as chief leadership officer to someone else, thereby denying himself followers.

Focus the assessment on the deeper dimensions of potential followers. Unfortunately, in assessments, titled executives look at organizational artifacts such as policies, procedures, and plans, even though written policies and procedures are no guarantee of organizational effectiveness. It is people on whom an assessment should concentrate. Even the Joint Commission on Accreditation of Healthcare Organizations has focused some of its attention on organizational intangibles such as leadership, mission, and change management.

Treat assessment as an ongoing program—not just a component of the annual performance appraisal. In most industries, people are assessed in annual evaluations that have more to do with anniversary dates than with behavior and performance. Typically, during annual evaluations the principle of recency dominates: People are often evaluated on the basis of the accomplishments they recorded and the mistakes they made in the 30 days immediately before the evaluation. Also, titled executives many times feel compelled to find something wrong with their employees. No one could be that good, they reason. There's no such thing as a very superior rating. As a result, titled executives often dish out an equal measure of carrots and sticks as incentives and are not able to consistently inspire followers.

In the worst case, these annual evaluations are anti-followership because they deflate and demotivate employees. If you find this hard to believe, answer this question: When was the last time an annual evaluation motivated you to greater productivity and excellence? Ask the same question of your colleagues, and you will probably discover that evaluations often diminish enthusiasm. Not only does preevaluation anxiety reduce productivity but, in many cases, employees will be tortured by self-doubts after an evaluation: Why am I here? What am I doing? I'm giving the best years of my life to this organization, and what am I getting in return?

During an annual evaluation, a nursing director was told, "Some people around here don't think you're a very good manager." "What do you mean?" she asked. "Give me some examples." "Well, I really can't say," the superior replied. "I just want you to know that there's a perception." After the evaluation, the director felt as though she had been torpedoed. Unfortunately, her attitude toward herself, her peers, and her work came to be shaped almost exclusively by such vague and non-behaviorally specific comments.

Consider the manager of dietary services who is verbally drawn and quartered in his vice president's office, only to have the VP smile and say, "We really like having you around here." If workers are labeled good one day and bad the next, or if they are labeled as both good and bad in the same conversation, what will they believe, and whom will they trust? Can they ever follow their boss? Bewildered and irritated, these employees typically become less effective in their jobs and avoid contact with their unpredictable superiors.

What, then, is the ideal? A healthy organization prepares people to *engage* in self-evaluation and self-motivation immediately on their hire dates. It is made clear to them that behavior A is productive and valuable to the organization, whereas behavior B is destructive and should be avoided. In this scheme, annual evaluations become nothing more than a sum of the many periodic evaluations and a forum to prepare goals for the coming year.

Reassure your followers. Followers need support. Followers need feedback. They need permission to express their beliefs in person, in e-mail, or on paper with no fear of reprisal. When an organizational assessment is scheduled, leaders realize that people may be on the defensive. They take the time to let people know that they understand the reasons for their defensiveness. Most importantly, leaders make it clear to followers that the purpose of assessment is not to weed out undesirables. The reason of the assessment is to focus the purpose of the organization and the work values of the employees. Given a clear purpose, the roles and contributions of employees can be clarified. Followers will respond with enthusiasm.

Distinguish assessment and evaluation from each other. Assessment involves the collection of data, whereas evaluation involves judgment. In most cases, judgments, decisions, statements, and evaluations should be buttressed by data, evidence, and supporting material.

Suspend judgment until the context is clear. Even when the data have been gathered, judgment on the organization must still be made carefully and in context. Despite the claims of pop management books, there are no good or bad cultures. In World War II, General George Patton created a highly effective culture for the mission he had to accomplish. However, his leadership style was inappropriate during peace time. In the same way, Mother Teresa inspired the most effective culture for her mission. Both General Patton and Mother Teresa are regarded as highly successful, charismatic leaders, but they had fundamentally different missions and thus different followers. Cultures, therefore, are neither inherently good nor bad. (Some organizations, however, can become pathological, toxic, and destructive usually because of an underground network of subcultures that wage war with each other.) Through the assessment process, data can be collected on the strength of the organization's culture. Judgment and planning must be reserved until the context for evaluation is clear.

"We have used the strategic planning process to help followers understand their roles in what we are trying to accomplish. Their involvement in the planning process increases their commitment to success."

—Raymond V. Ingham, PH.D., FACHE, president and CEO, Witham Health Services, Lebanon, Indiana

Determine and convey the role of the assessor and the person being assessed early on. The roles of those who are to be assessed and those who are to use the data need to be identified. There must also be a clear understanding of who will design the assessment instrument, who will make decisions about the questions, who will receive the survey, and who will ultimately define the context to judge the data.

Make sure the assessment is conducted and processed objectively by outside facilitators. It is very difficult to administer an assessment of the intangibles in one's own organization. Is the president of a financially troubled organization really the best person to lead a management/board retreat on turnaround strategies? Unfortunately, many titled executives are slow to accept the necessity of consultants who deal with human capital. They pay $300 to $500 per hour to attorneys without a second thought; they bring in accountants when only a minor variation is uncovered in financial statements. When a new building is needed, few executives sit down on the weekend with a book on architectural design. Nevertheless, these same executives often assume that they can easily understand the most complicated dynamic of any organization—human motivation.

Ask yourself why you are doing the assessment. Leaders always ask what their personal motivations are for conducting the assessment. Inevitably they will ask, Why are we doing this anyway? Some form of this answer must be forthcoming. Leaders use assessments to communicate a need to learn from followers about how to improve the workplace environment.

All other barriers to assessment must be confronted with similar openness. As mentioned before, many titled executives hold back on assessment out of fear of what it may uncover. As one cautious CEO asked, "What if I find out that morale is low?" But an assessment tool would do nothing more than quantify the situation so that he could take action. Unfortunately, some titled executives prefer to serve as caretakers of dysfunctional and toxic organizations rather than confront the truth and do the hard work needed to manage change by increasing followership.

Assessment is admittedly difficult. It means that the government, physicians, fluoridated water, insurance companies, Wall Street, the crumbling public educational system, or some other societal element can no longer be blamed. The fact is that the destiny of an organization and its people is in the leader's hands. In the course of an assessment it may even be discovered that the reluctance to assess the organization is rooted in the titled executive's philosophy of human nature. If so, she must be brutally frank with herself. Does she believe that people need to be whipped or they will not perform well? Does she see employees as little more than interchangeable parts in the profit process? Does she look on theories about human capital as mindless drivel?

In sum, data collection tools, as well as the spirit or attitude with which the assessment is conducted, should be approached cautiously. Most of all, every effort should be made to turn what could be a boring, tedious schoolroom exercise into an opportunity. Quite simply, conducting an assessment should be seen as a way to produce a more effective organization through engagement and alignment of followers.

SAMPLE ASSESSMENT TOOL BASED ON PERSONAL INVESTMENT VALUES

Once the organization is ready to begin the assessment process, it must choose an appropriate instrument. There are many excellent instruments available to healthcare leaders today. The instrument featured here contains material from the Healthcare Organizational Assessment Survey designed by MetriTech, Inc. (Braskamp and Maehr 1986, 37).* This 200-item survey uses *The Motivational Factor: A Theory of Personal Investment* (Maehr and

---

* Copyright © 1985 by MetriTech, Inc., Champaign, IL. Reproduced by permission.

Braskamp 1986) as the basis for its design. It assesses the four values of personal investment—recognition, accomplishment, power, and affiliation—according to how people perceive themselves, their jobs, and the organization.

Recognition

Person: How important are financial rewards and acknowledgments from others?
Job: Do employees receive extra benefits for doing good work?
Organization: Do people believe the organization does a good job of rewarding the achievements and contributions of its employees?

If recognition is a strong value, people will respond positively to the following statements:

- Employees in this organization receive a lot of attention.
- In this organization, they make me feel like a winner.
- This organization allows me to do those things that I find personally satisfying.
- There are many incentives to work hard.

Accomplishment

Person: How much do people strive for excellence, and how much do they enjoy and value challenging and exciting work?
Job: To what extent do they strive for excellence in what they do? Is this job an exciting and challenging one?
Organization: Does this organization emphasize excellence in products and services?

If accomplishment is a strong value in your organization, people will respond positively to the following statements:

- I am encouraged to make suggestions about how we can be more effective.
- Around here, we are encouraged to try new things.
- In this organization, we are given a great deal of freedom to carry out our work.
- If someone has a good idea, invention, or project, management will listen and support it.

Power

Person: To what degree do employees compete with one another to gain authority and to advance within the organization?
Job: Can I influence others through this job?
Organization: Does this organization create an environment in which conflict and competition are assumed and expected?

If power is a strong value in your organization, people will respond positively to the following statements:

- Successful people are those who like to win.
- I emerged as the leader of my group.
- People seek me out for advice.
- Competition among different work groups is actively encouraged.

Affiliation

Person: How important are showing concern and affection to others and making sacrifices to help others develop?
Job: Does this job help others?
Organization: Is the organization one that emphasizes mutual support, open communication, sharing of information, and caring for each individual?

If affiliation is a strong value, people will respond positively to the following statements:

- In this organization, they really care about me as a person.
- We are treated like adults in this organization.
- In this organization, there is respect for each individual worker.
- I am involved in decisions that directly affect my work in this organization.

As shown above, the focus of each of the four values should be on the person, the job, and the organization. To assess these three factors, employees should be asked to respond to the following series of statements by noting if they (1) strongly agree, (2) agree, (3) are uncertain, (4) disagree, or (5) strongly disagree.

The first set of questions is meant to elicit information about the personality of the employee.

> "Followers want to see the leader as a good person who is concerned about the follower's development. Leaders need to listen, disclose some things about themselves in order to engage followers."
>
> —*Vicki L. Romero, president and CEO, Longview Regional Medical Center, Longview, Texas*

- I enjoy completing many easy tasks rather than just a few difficult ones.
- I pay little attention to the interests of people around me.
- I want recognition for what I do.
- I emerged as a leader in my group.

In a similar way, employees' reactions to their present job or position in the organization can be evaluated by asking them to choose an answer that completes the following statement:

My present job provides opportunities
- to show my competence and ability.
- to help people directly.

- to receive recognition for my work.
- to hire and fire employees.

Finally, it can be determined how people feel about the organization by asking them to react to the following statements:

- My coworkers and I work well together.
- I feel I get sufficient pay for the work I do.
- I have the opportunity to do good work here and thus advance myself.
- I have a sense of loyalty to this place.

OUTCOME MEASUREMENTS

Responses to these and similar questions provide three outcome measurements—strength of culture, job satisfaction, and organizational commitment—which together form the bottom line of human capital.

Strength of Culture

The strength of the culture can be viewed as the balance sheet on the intangibles. How strong is the organization's culture? What does the intangible's balance sheet look like? Do employees believe that the organization has done a good job of defining and communicating its mission? Do they see the organization as having a clear sense of direction (vision)? Do people understand what is expected of them (values)? If the culture is strong, employees see their organization as having a clear set of norms and a strong sense of direction. They know what the organization stands for and what really counts. Agreement on values is pervasive and deep. Each follower has a strong sense of ownership in what happens around him or her.

Job Satisfaction

Job satisfaction reflects the profit/loss ratio on the intangibles. What are the short-term good and bad aspects of working here? What is the current climate? How satisfied are people with their work, pay, promotion opportunities, supervision, and coworkers? When people experience job satisfaction, they answer the question Do you enjoy your job? with an emphatic yes. If people are committed to an organization, they tend to enjoy their job, but it does not necessarily follow that someone who is satisfied with his or her job is committed to the organization. Although satisfaction might not predict commitment, commitment predicts satisfaction.

Organizational Commitment

Commitment may be seen as the net worth of the intangibles. When the negatives are subtracted from the positives, what is left? Viewed another way, commitment—not satisfaction—predicts retention, and commitment comes from shared values, meaning, loyalty, pride, and ownership. Hospitals with strong cultures enjoy high levels of commitment among their workers. When followers commit themselves to an organization, they believe in it and understand it. Only when an organization has a defined mission, internalized values, and a clear vision are employees likely to say, "Now that we understand what we're about, we know how we fit in and we won't leave here."

Culture, commitment, and satisfaction can be analyzed for the organization as well as for distinct subgroups within it—for example, the senior management team, board members, medical staff leadership, department heads, and support staff. Total organizational scores provide a good starting point, but viewing the scores according to subgroups will both pinpoint areas of strength that can be used to better the organization and identify those weaknesses that may require special attention when instituting any kind of managed change program.

ASSESSING LEADERSHIP SKILLS

The period just after completion of the organizational assessment may be the perfect time for leaders to further assess their leadership skills. Leaders should rate themselves on the issues of structure, feedback, productivity, failure, accountability, communication, ownership, reward, and values. Questions related to each of these issues are listed below. In each case they should describe their typical behaviors and actions as well as how followers are affected by them. A leader should pose two questions: (1) What is my standard operating procedure? and (2) Does it increase or decrease followership?

Structure. How is work structured? Does the structure liberate people and make them more productive, or does it constrain and demoralize people?

Feedback. What kind of feedback do people receive? In what form and through what vehicles? To what extent is the feedback constructive, positive, and motivating? To what extent is it negative? How often do you hear people say, "You never get a thank you around here. They never appreciate what you do"? To what degree are people affected by the absence of positive feedback? Are you guilty of delivering mixed messages that confuse and traumatize people?

Productivity. How is productivity defined and measured in this organization? To what extent am I guilty of a desire to reduce all performance to standards that no one disagrees with? Are individuals who can produce financial gains or cost savings rewarded more consistently than those who make significant intangible contributions? What is the organization's concept of a "productive employee," and how does that person differ from a "busy employee"?

Failure. To what extent does this organization encourage risk taking and tolerate—even accept—failure? How are people encouraged to take risks? What kinds of safety nets or parachutes are provided? When people failed in the past, how were they treated? How are people treated when they succeed?

Accountability. How are people held accountable for their performance? To what extent are people given clear expectations as well as opportunities to "stretch"? Are people allowed to pass the buck and blame others for their failures, or is self-management the norm?

Communication. When decisions are made, how are they shared with the organization? To what extent are people given the opportunity for serious input? Is criticism tolerated and even encouraged? Or are outspoken employees punished as disruptive troublemakers? How are disputes or conflicts resolved? Is silence interpreted as compliance/support?

Ownership. To what extent do people feel invested in the organization? Are they able to decide independently and take action, or do they always have to appeal to higher authority? How are autonomy and personal growth encouraged? To what extent are people encouraged to give positive feedback to themselves and others? Or do people depend exclusively on their superiors or on financial rewards for validation of self-worth?

Reward. How are rewards contingent on values-based behavior? Are high-performing people often rewarded through promotions and compensation? Are they rewarded for values-based, mission-driven, and team-oriented behavior? Or are rewards mainly given to hard-nosed bottom-line contributors? Can I balance rewards for both tangible and intangible behavior?

Values. Are values instilled at all levels of this organization? If so, through what vehicles? Do people understand the values of this organization and how they can be translated into behavior? Are the values felt "in the gut"?

Unfortunately, many instruments designed to assess leadership measure only satisfiers and dissatisfiers. Independent of an organization's context, satisfiers mean little. Many healthcare executives who have risen to top spots in religious institutions would probably be uncomfortable in investor-owned systems. In the same way, an aggressive, financially oriented MBA might grow frustrated and impatient with an organization that begins each day in meditation and prayer. Although these executives might have similar academic credentials, their behavior is driven by different beliefs and values.

Leadership theories often focus solely on what leaders do and ignore what potential followers need. This is a mistake. Leadership must concern itself both with actions and the impact of those actions on others. Leadership involves not only action and quantifiable results but also the spirit that is developed and built among followers. Leadership is more than a matter of new and better programs and services; it also encompasses the values and beliefs that are integrated into new projects. Leadership is about followership. Leadership starts with what a person does and ends with the effects of those actions on the people who are expected to follow.

All too often, executives embrace the latest best-selling business book as a cure for their own organization's ills. Although they see promise in the maneuvers of a Herb Kelleher, a Sam Walton, or a Jack Welch (the men who made successes of Southwest Airlines, Wal-Mart, and General Electric, respectively), they often discover that imitation—while it may be a sincere form of flattery—usually has limited impact. As the fumbling successor to the CEO of a major healthcare system once said, "I don't know what's wrong. I'm doing everything she did." In making that statement, he was missing a crucial point: Plans, procedures, and policies were essential ingredients to his predecessor's success, but even more important were her values and the spirit infused in her followers.

Consider the titled healthcare executive who has read every book published on leadership in the last five years. He understands the magic of one-minute interactions, management by walking around, moving cheese, blowing everything up, and even throwing fish. Although he appears to do everything right, nothing works. Why? Because he never assimilated the philosophies and principles that undergird innovative organizations and drive leaders. He uses all the right words and gestures, but no one believes him. As a result, he has no followers.

Leadership is a byproduct of what a person believes about those whom she wants to turn into followers. If she looks on these individuals as valuable human beings and effective workers with unlimited potential, her role will become that of facilitator, servant, enabler. A leader's task is to create followers by making them feel positive about themselves, their performance, and the organization. A leader views people as partners and associates in a collective quest.

The ultimate goals of assessment are self-monitoring and ownership of behavior (accountability). A person who is unable to monitor himself or herself necessarily depends on outside authority for direction. "I don't know what to do" is the typical response to any decision-making opportunity, "I'll talk to my boss." In organizations with strong leadership, something

> "Performing an inventory assessment of the organization and of the healthcare executive is of vital importance to the future survival of the organization. We must continually scrutinize our personal leadership style to ensure our continued effectiveness throughout the organization."
>
> —Michael Rust, FACHE, president and CEO, Kentucky Hospital Association, Louisville, Kentucky

else happens. Every follower in the organization—regardless of position—learns to make decisions that benefit the organization because the followers know what the organization stands for and how they fit. They feel confident and have access to the information necessary to make decisions consistent with the aims of the organization. Confident that failure will not result in painful reprisals, followers feel free to disregard the limitations of a specific job description.

Self-managed, motivated followers communicate their enthusiasm for their work and their organization. Such people live the principles of service, safety, and quality. And today, service, patient safety, and quality are the difference between success and failure in healthcare.

REFERENCES

Braskamp, L. A., and M. L. Maehr. 1986. The Healthcare Organizational Assessment Survey. Champaign, IL: MetriTech, Inc.

Collins, J. 2001. *Good to Great: Why Some Companies Make the Leap . . . and Others Don't.* New York: HarperCollins.

Maehr, M., and L. Braskamp. 1986. *The Motivation Factor: A Theory of Personal Investment.* Lanham, MD: Lexington Books.

CHAPTER 7

Analysis:
Focusing on Increasing Followership

LEADERS UNDERSTAND THAT raw data must be converted to meaningful information to inspire followers. Interpretation and judgment provide the bridge between assessment and analysis, between data and information. Interpretation means describing the data in specific, concrete, and objective terms. For example, "motivation is increasing in operations by 3.2 percent compared to last quarter," "satisfaction is 1.5 percent down in the emergency department compared to last month," or "commitment is up by 2.6 percent with the cardiac surgeons." Interpretation tells us what the numbers say. Judgment tells us how fast we can go, how much we can expect, and so on in the context of the overall vision/goal/objectives.

Analysis is fundamentally different from assessment. During assessment, behavior is converted into numbers. In analysis, leaders try to evaluate those numbers. Analysis is nothing more than judging the numbers to be "good" or "bad." If you discover that your blood pressure is 190 over 150, it means little until your physician tells you, "That's high." The physician has analyzed the numbers, given them meaning, and made a judgment. Leadership requires you to accept the responsibility of evaluation and to help staff understand the context of your decisions—that is, what are the decision rules?

Typically, analysis makes use of words such as *good, reliable, effective,* and *worthwhile.* Evaluation is evident in the statements, "Our greatest asset is our nursing staff," "This survey received a better response rate than the last one," "The level of participation in that program is disappointing," and "Morale is low this month." All of these statements involve judgments based on data. They go beyond a description of what is occurring to an assertion of whether something is good or bad, harmful or beneficial, negative or positive. Leaders always anchor judgments in the organization's culture. Remember, there are no good or bad cultures (only clashing subcultures), and judgments about goodness or badness can only be made in the context of the corporate culture, especially the values. Judging data in context is the essence of analysis and your key function as a healthcare leader committed to organizational change. Culture-based analysis is the foundation of all managed change programs. Consistent, values-based decisions will attract and sustain those followers who share your values.

> "The leader must crystallize the framework for all decisions. Followers know that 'A' is more important than 'B.' This framework is best built by being 'out there,' by being present."
>
> —Mark Taylor, president and CEO, St. John's Hospital, Detroit, Michigan

EFFECTIVE ORGANIZATIONS

The effective healthcare organization is characterized by five factors:

1. high quality
2. high employee and physician commitment
3. high patient satisfaction (which includes patient safety)
4. high market share
5. high profit

When these factors are present, the culture is strong, the business factors are good, change is being managed well, and there is a good sense of teamwork. The more effective your organization, the more these factors will increase. However, if you notice that quality, commitment, patient satisfaction, profit, and market share are on the downswing, you will want to introduce the following general questions: How do we become a more effective organization? What aspect of our culture changed, and why? Why did commitment weaken? Did the organization fail to offer enough rewards and recognition to good employees? Why do followers feel less attached to their boss? All answers to ineffectiveness lie in the analysis of the intangibles.

Take time out to analyze the effectiveness of your organization by asking the targeted questions that follow:

- How personally invested are your employees? What assessment data are you using in your analysis? Are there reasons to be concerned about their level of commitment?
- What are the most effective parts of your organization? What is driving the corporate culture and the business's success? In which areas are best practices for the tangibles and intangibles being exhibited?
- Is your vision of the organization clear to your employees? Are followers inspired by the direction you are taking the company? Have you communicated and clarified their role in achieving this direction?
- How successful will you be in achieving your tangible objectives with the intangible (motivational) aspects revealed by your assessment?
- How would you change your followership profile? What traits or behaviors would be ideal for the support staff, medical staff, board or trustees, professional staff, and management team? For example, would you want the organization to become more risk taking and entrepreneurial? Would you

want more teamwork and bottom-up decision making to take place?

- If you need to strengthen your culture, what values should you emphasize in all of your analysis and decision making?

Financial audits are used to identify business strengths and weaknesses. In a very similar way, cultural audits are used to isolate effective practices that correspond to the values of the organization and to identify the areas that must be emphasized if a positive corporate culture and profitable business ventures are to be maintained. The leader must bring all of these assessment and analysis factors to bear when developing a plan of action. The following section provides a complete list of the audit factors to be used in identifying areas of change.

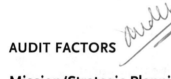

AUDIT FACTORS

Mission/Strategic Planning

1. We have a long-range vision that we continually use in planning.
2. We use our core values as the main basis for hiring new people.
3. We engage our followers in all goal discussions.
4. We discuss our mission statement at all goal-revision sessions.
5. We spend more time on long-range plans than on short-term solutions.

Socialization

1. I often hear stories about the contributions of our followers.
2. This organization is never dull or unexciting.

3. Leaders in the organization know how to inspire followers.
4. We have social events in which we celebrate our accomplishments.
5. Mentors take a new person to lunch on his or her first day at work.
6. We have parties to help new employees get to know their peers better.
7. We recognize special events such as birthdays.
8. I often hear others speak of our organization as one big family.
9. We reward high performers constantly.

> "To be truly outstanding requires a disciplined approach towards focusing on what is relevant for the organization to succeed."
>
> —*Wayne Lerner*, DR.P.H., FACHE, *president and* CEO, *Rehabilitation Institute of Chicago*

Selection

1. People who work here must go through a thorough screening process that determines whether their personal values match corporate values.
2. Job roles and expectations are made explicit to each applicant.
3. Teamwork expectations are explained to screen out anyone who would not work well with others.
4. We have a very low tolerance for poor performers.

Standards/Expectations

1. Expectations about what and how much employees will have to do are negotiated by leaders with followers.
2. All followers are able to see how their goals help achieve the vision of the organization.
3. The organization has clear standards of performance, and

those who do not meet them are first helped with extra training.

4. If, after help, an employee does not meet corporate values and business-based expectations, he or she is released from the organization.

5. If the expectations held by followers and leaders do not align, we feel free to discuss the problem openly.

Performance Appraisal

1. All followers work with their leaders to define how to perform their duties and what they should be accomplishing.

2. Leaders provide routine and frequent feedback.

3. All followers are engaged in a process to determine how much they are to accomplish.

4. Followers say that they get enough relevant and immediate information on how well they are doing.

5. Evaluation of work is very informal and frequent.

6. Evaluation about whether promotion is needed is values based.

7. Evaluation of work always includes discussion about how to improve and what organizational support is available for professional development.

Teamwork

1. Leaders and followers structure goals so that they can work together in teams.

2. Groups are rewarded as a unit when they are successful.

3. Groups share the responsibility of determining how to proceed to get work done.

4. We think in terms of group projects rather than individual assignments.

Participation in Management

1. The lines of authority in this organization are clear but not rigid or autocratic.
2. Everyone in the organization can take on almost any role because titles and positions are defined by what is needed to succeed.
3. Before we make a decision or establish a policy, everyone who will be affected is consulted.
4. Followers' participation in decision making is very high.
5. Many people review designs and plans before we implement them.
6. We hold special retreats to discuss the future of our organization.
7. Expectations for performance in this organization are clearly defined.
8. Rules and regulations are values based and internalized.
9. Our formal rules and regulations never get in the way of patient safety and satisfaction. We believe in the phrase "Whatever it takes!"
10. We are known as a company with very little bureaucracy, high performers, and satisfied customers.

Communication Networks

1. Leadership promotes open communication among all units of the organization.
2. Staff meetings are held as needed. No meeting is held without a clear benefit to all attending.
3. Communication in the organization is very informal.
4. House organs are used to communicate best practices.
5. All leaders have an open-door policy.
6. Followers can go around their immediate supervisor to solve a problem.

7. Upper-level leadership sponsors lunches and open meetings to hear the concerns of the followers.

improvement

Career Succession/Advancement

1. Everyone is in charge of his or her own future in this organization.
2. Followers are encouraged to grow professionally and to become better team players.
3. There are many avenues for advancement in this organization.
4. Career counseling and advice are available.
5. Everyone can talk confidentially with those in human resources about the probability of advancing in the organization.
6. We have created our own "leadership development institute."

> "'Little things mean a lot' is our motto for change. We measure and analyze all meaningful ways to help staff (followers) to improve their effectiveness."
>
> —*Kelly Mather, CEO, Sutter Lakeside Hospital, Lakeport, California*

Organizational Adaptability

1. This organization makes changes quickly to meet increasing demands.
2. Everyone is very concerned about how others view our services.
3. We are continually doing market surveys to learn how to best meet the wants and needs of our customers, patients, and physicians.
4. We are continually experimenting with new programs and approaches to make our services better.
5. We are encouraged to take risks.

6. We work closely with all our customer groups so that we can provide services that fit their needs and wants.
7. We are concerned about how our best clients view us.
8. We make it a point to listen carefully to what our customers want from us.

Organizational Structure

1. We believe in adaptability and thus are always ready to refocus our human and financial capital to meet market opportunities and customer needs.
2. We have a flat arrangement of positions and roles within the organization characterized by little bureaucracy, few layers of management, and decision making by those serving customers.
3. In this organization, followers are put into small units that have the freedom to do things in ways that best meet patient, physician, and other customer needs.
4. In this organization the emphasis is on keeping the work units small and flexible.
5. To solve special problems and/or test innovative ideas, we establish informal ad hoc task forces.
6. Every person in the organization is free to suggest new ideas and solutions to problems.
7. We emphasize the importance of each role within a team and spell out what is expected of the person in that role.

Recognition Practices

1. We have a parking spot for the employee of the month.
2. We have recognition dinners at least once a year.
3. We publish the pictures of those named employee of the month.

4. We have a policy of writing letters and notes to those who have done outstanding work.
5. There is a section in our house organ (in-house newsletter, etc.) that deals with recognition of employees.
6. All rewards are based on team contributions to achieving the organization's vision within the context of our core values. (For more detail on the difference between rewards and recognition, see Atchison 2003.)

Financial Incentives/Salary Program

1. Exceptional individuals and teams can get bonuses.
2. Salary increases are based on team performance rather than on longevity.

MAXIMIZING EFFECTIVENESS: ESSENTIALS

Behavioral audits of all relationships and dynamics are used to show the causes of and barriers to building committed followers. Behavioral audits also show the variances in the strength of the organization's culture among different work groups. These variances will pinpoint areas where managed change is most feasible. It should be reiterated that there are no absolute right or wrong analyses. The important thing is to define those values-based behaviors that the organization emphasizes and to determine where followers are most in harmony with them.

Here are the essentials that must be measured and analyzed to maximize organizational performance. A strong culture exists when (1) followers view the organization as having a clear set of values and a sense of direction, (2) follower values and organizational values converge, (3) commitment is high and jobs are challenging, (4) followers work cooperatively to achieve the organization's vision because they feel ownership of and pride in the success of the organization, (5) followers are encouraged to take risks and are rewarded for contributions to their team, and (6) the emphasis is on the development of the human capital of the organization.

A CASE STUDY: AFFINITY HEALTH SYSTEM

The corporate office for Affinity Health System (AHS) is located in Menasha, Wisconsin. Affinity Health System resulted from a 1997 merger of Mercy Hospital in Oshkosh and St. Elizabeth Hospital in Appleton, both in Wisconsin. The merger also included a large medical group, an insurance company, and several community clinics. The two parent companies are the Wheaton Franciscans and the Ministry Health Care, both of which share equally in governance.

> "In a world of 'profitless growth,' the key to success lies in the degree to which the leader can motivate the staff. That is, how many will follow you?"
>
> —Raymond V. Ingham, PH.D., FACHE, president and CEO, Witham Health Services, Lebanon, Indiana

Kevin Nolan became the president and CEO in March 1999. His first task was to create a strong AHS corporate culture. He began with the hiring of Debbie Grogan-Wood as the senior vice president of human resources. They needed some baseline data and completed an assessment of AHS's corporate culture in November 1999. The data from the initial assessment are displayed in Table 7.1.

The data showed an organization that was floundering, without direction, and dominated by suspicion and mistrust. Any score for the three culture factors—commitment, satisfaction, and strength of culture—above 75 percent is very good; any score below 25 percent is very weak. AHS's level of commitment of 63 percent is considered a good score. This level of commitment shows that the senior staff had a slightly higher than average sense of loyalty and pride. The low job satisfaction score of 34 percent

Table 7.1: AHS 1999 Organizational Assessment Analysis Grid, Total Group (*N* = 122)

	Influence		
Value Stressed	*Person*	*Job*	*Organization*
Recognition	39	59	20
Accomplishment	35	56	52
Power	14	71	91
Affiliation	94	70	15

Commitment	Satisfaction	Strength of Culture
63	34	7

shows a group of senior managers who were worried about their job and felt stressed and uncertain about the future. AHS's strength-of-culture score of 7 percent is very low.

In 1999, AHS had no common culture. This describes an organization that is not aware of its purpose, its direction, or the core values that underpin decisions. Organizations with essentially no corporate culture behave in any way that allows each unit to protect its "territory." Without an overriding corporate culture, organizations default to survival, skepticism, and resistance. These were the behaviors that most described AHS in 1999. The dynamics of the work environment were further complicated by the fact that Nolan and Grogan-Wood were brought into AHS from the outside. They were, in fact, viewed as "outsiders" who did not understand that "this is the way we always did it."

Assessment is a prerequisite to alignment of the leader's vision and the followers' trust. Without data, we all default to subjectivity. Clearly communicated valid and reliable data are an important building block in the leader-follower relationship.

The data for the total AHS leadership group are displayed in Table 7.2. Subgroup data are presented in Tables 7.3, 7.4, and 7.5. The analysis of these data drove specific interventions for the AHS system as well as subgroups. The main motivational influences of recognition, accomplishment, power, and affiliation were measured for all major leadership groups (Figure 7.1). The data show a very caring group (i.e., high affiliation scores) who has little motivation to take risks or deal with conflict (i.e., low power scores). This pattern of high affiliation and low power is very common in healthcare. This pattern combined with initial low scores on strength of culture and job satisfaction (Figure 7.2) required AHS executives not only to analyze ways to improve but also to decide what pattern of intangibles is best to achieve the vision.

Nolan, AHS's president and CEO, realized the depth of the problem. He recognized that there was no easy, piecemeal fix to the multiple dimensions contributing to these low scores, and he decided that a complete cultural transformation was needed. The five different entities making up AHS had five different agendas and were supported by five different subcultures. There was no trust among the entities, no sense of collaboration, a great deal of internal competition, and essentially no system-focused communication. These cultural dynamics drove a weak business profile: AHS lost $13,437,000 in fiscal year 1999 and $15,151,000 in fiscal year 2000 (Figure 7.3).

Nolan began by retooling and aligning his executive team. He added high-performing, system-focused professionals, and he mentored those who were already in place to become more innovative. Along with his chief medical officer, Scott Nygaard, M.D., they began the difficult job of developing a physician leadership council. The human resources senior vice president, Grogan-Wood, created a cultural change team called the "Guiding Coalition."

The benefits of this multifaceted approach to transforming the corporate culture are reflected in the 2002 assessment data

Table 7.2: AHS **Organizational Assessment Analysis Grid, Total Group**

Value Stressed	Influence		
	Person	Job	Organization
Recognition			
2002 — N = 129	62	78	65
2001 — N = 130	30	75	41
1999 — N = 122	39	59	20
Accomplishment			
2002 — N = 129	55	71	85
2001 — N = 130	40	69	70
1999 — N = 122	35	56	52
Power			
2002 — N = 129	24	77	86
2001 — N = 130	21	77	90
1999 — N = 122	14	71	91
Affiliation			
2002 — N = 129	95	82	75
2001 — N = 130	94	79	41
1999 — N = 122	94	70	15

Year	Commitment	Satisfaction	Strength of Culture
2002 — N = 129	78	64	72
2001 — N = 130	58	50	23
1999 — N = 122	63	34	7

(see Tables 7.2 to 7.5) and the financial improvement (see Figure 7.3). AHS has also received recognition as the 11th-highest-rated integrated health network by *Modern Healthcare* (Lauer et al. 2002).

Nolan (2003) says that his job now is to set strategic goals and create an environment that unleashes the talents and skills of all

Table 7.3: AHS **Organizational Assessment Analysis Grid, Executive Team**

Value Stressed	Influence		
	Person	Job	Organization
Recognition			
2002 — $N = 12$	16	100	97
2001 — $N = 15$	22	98	65
1999 — $N = 15$	14	94	44
Accomplishment			
2002 — $N = 12$	96	96	96
2001 — $N = 15$	64	82	80
1999 — $N = 15$	44	96	69
Power			
2002 — $N = 12$	82	96	99
2001 — $N = 15$	84	90	95
1999 — $N = 15$	57	88	95
Affiliation			
2002 — $N = 12$	99	97	98
2001 — $N = 15$	79	91	64
1999 — $N = 15$	96	95	43

Year	Commitment	Satisfaction	Strength of Culture
2002 — $N = 12$	97	100	99
2001 — $N = 15$	70	80	69
1999 — $N = 15$	93	84	46

"the marvelous people who care for our patients. We are now pulling in the same direction to deliver high-quality care to this community." Nolan transformed the AHS culture by selecting high-performing professionals who are committed to live the values as they achieve the mission and vision.

Table 7.4: AHS Organizational Assessment Analysis Grid, Department Directors

Value Stressed	Influence		
	Person	Job	Organization
Recognition			
2002 — N = 43	53	86	72
2001 — N = 41	36	82	55
1999 — N = 47	39	59	20
Accomplishment			
2002 — N = 43	71	82	88
2001 — N = 41	44	74	69
1999 — N = 47	70	72	56
Power			
2002 — N = 43	43	80	92
2001 — N = 41	26	81	91
1999 — N = 47	15	68	88
Affiliation			
2002 — N = 43	89	85	83
2001 — N = 41	90	81	50
1999 — N = 47	91	73	20
Year	Commitment	Satisfaction	Strength of Culture
2002 — N = 43	80	88	87
2001 — N = 41	48	57	28
1999 — N = 47	65	55	5

THE LEADERSHIP PROCESS FOR MANAGING CHANGE

The structured process of staff assessment, analysis of data, and review of audits paved the way for a very successful managed change program at AHS, as shown by the high post-assessment scores. The principles of the leadership process used by Nolan and his team

Table 7.5: AHS **Organizational Assessment Analysis Grid, Department Managers**

	Influence		
Value Stressed	Person	Job	Organization
Recognition			
2002 — N = 79	69	68	59
2001 — N = 72	29	58	30
1999 — N = 57	41	48	13
Accomplishment			
2002 — N = 79	47	62	82
2001 — N = 72	34	61	69
1999 — N = 57	13	34	44
Power			
2002 — N = 79	17	75	82
2001 — N = 72	11	73	87
1999 — N = 57	6	69	93
Affiliation			
2002 — N = 79	97	80	68
2001 — N = 72	97	74	32
1999 — N = 57	95	59	9

Year	Commitment	Satisfaction	Strength of Culture
2002 — N = 79	75	45	60
2001 — N = 72	61	39	15
1999 — N = 57	52	13	3

are described below. This same process has been used by other successful healthcare leaders throughout the country.

Using the Audits to Identify Areas for Change

AHS's uniformly low strength-of-culture scores, as discussed in the case study, indicated that the first order of business was to

Figure 7.1: AHS Total Group Motivational Scales

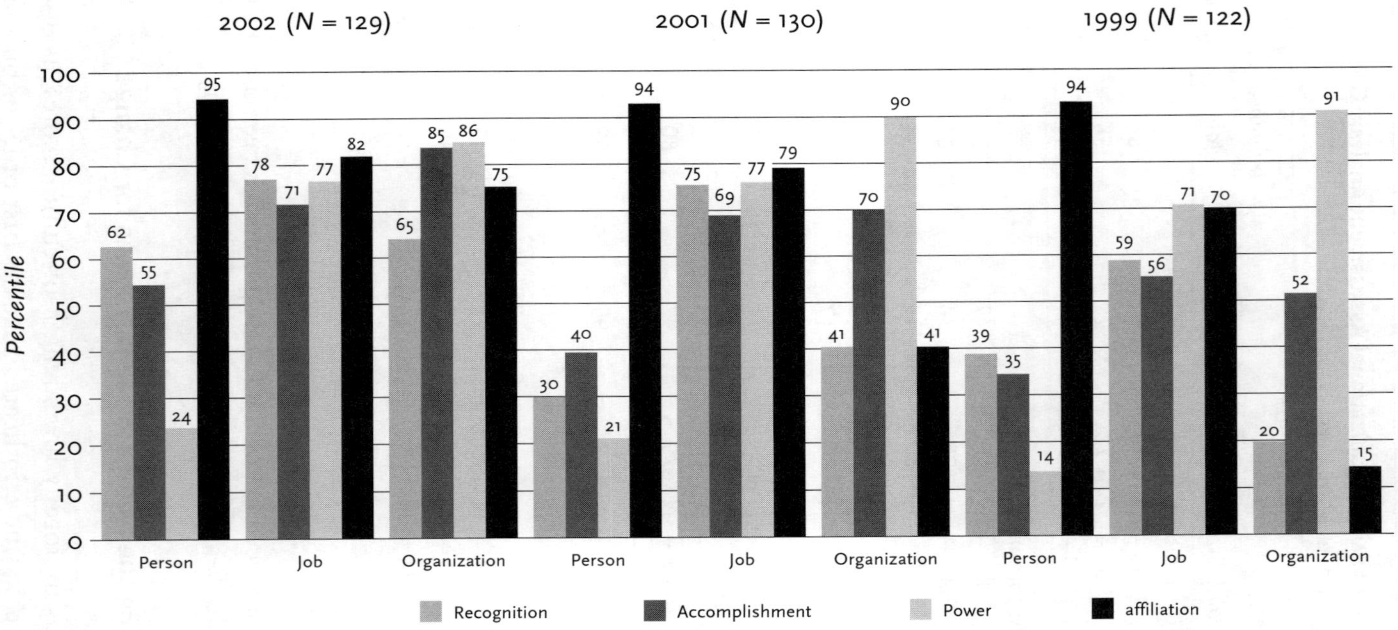

Figure 7.2: AHS Total Group Key Motivational Scales

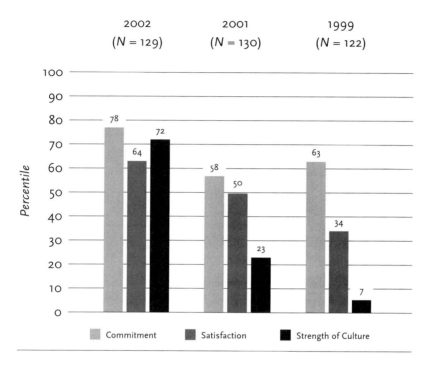

audit all statements relating to strength of culture and commitment. As a result of this audit process, AHS's Guiding Coalition decided that it needed to redefine the hospital's mission and values. In addition, managers audited all programs relating to recognition, accomplishment, and affiliation, paying particular attention to such matters as teamwork, participation in management, rewards and recognition, advancement, and performance appraisal.

Identifying the Barriers to Strengthening Your Culture

As you move from assessment to analysis, you must challenge the mission and values of your organization, but it is its vision that becomes the centerpiece, the pivot point on which you will make

Figure 7.3: AHS **Income from Operations (non-GAAP format)**

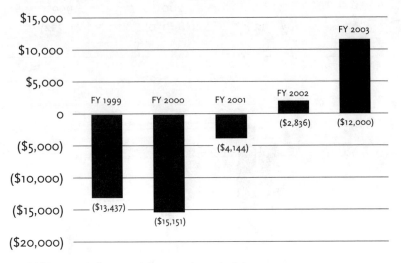

Note: GAAP = generally accepted accounting principles

your initial judgment. Take a quick inventory of your organization as documented in financial statements or marketing plans. Do you find evidence of increased bad debt, financial disappointments in new business ventures, retention problems among subspecialists, inadequate information systems, or a weak image among local businesses?

As a next step, overlay your vision statement on these data. To what extent does a problem identified here prevent you from achieving your vision? For example, suppose that part of your vision is to generate revenue through managed care contracts with local-area employers. Suppose further that the data reveal that you have employees who are high in the intangible factor of affiliation but low in accomplishment? They may be able to talk about the service, but can they do it without support? It will be difficult to achieve your vision with people who value support and caring more than financial success and the development of new linkages with local businesses. There is too great a disparity between corporate values and personal values. However, if your vision includes the healing tradition of a specific religious order, you may fall short with individuals who score high in power and low in affiliation.

In analyzing the fit of your mission with the values of the workforce, you should address several issues.

First, to what extent do your perceived problems touch on your vision? In light of your vision, what are your real problems or challenges? What trends should you be concerned about? On which people, situations, and events should you focus your attention and assets?

> "Everything must tie back to building trust. The importance of consistency, openness and predictability cannot be overstated."
>
> —*Vicki L. Romero, president and CEO, Longview Regional Medical Center, Longview, Texas*

Second, given the priorities identified in your vision statement, where do your followers stand? Do the data show that your workforce understands its role sufficiently to move the organization forward in the achievement of your vision? Or do the values profiles indicate that the organization may remain in a holding pattern or regress in the near future? To what extent is their understanding of what they contribute to the vision an indication that they would impede achievement of your goals?

Third, as an exercise, describe what the organization would be like if it were actively achieving its vision. How would it be different? Would the workforce as it currently exists be the same? How would its members need to change?

Fourth, summarize in what ways the dynamics of your workforce encourage the fulfillment of your overall vision and in what ways they tend to block it.

Analyzing Your Core Values: What Drives Your Decisions?

After analyzing your vision, look at your core beliefs. What convictions underpin choices in your organization? What is seen as most important? Is it respect for community support and teaching? Or is it opportunity, innovation, and excellence? After you have identified your values (the convictions that drive your decisions), examine what the data say about the values of your workforce. Once again, there may be conflicts between your organization's stated values and the operating values of your workforce.

In an organization that truly values caring and the dignity of the individual, people who have low affiliation scores and high power scores may face the classic problem of poor organizational fit. Why? Because if they are low in affiliation, they will probably never place much emphasis on caring for others. Therefore, people who value winning, success, and external recognition may find themselves at odds with an organization whose statement of philosophy refers to "vocation," "service," and "the noble act of caring." In analyzing values, ask the following questions:

1. What are the lived values of this organization—not just those that we pay lip service to? What do our behaviors say is most important?
2. To what extent does the values profile of our workforce complement or contradict our optimal organizational values profile?
3. What problems might result from a conflict in values? In contrast, what could be achieved if the values of the organization meshed with those of the workforce?
4. If a values conflict is uncovered, what are the options for dealing with it?

One CEO wanted to reinforce his organization's role in making the community a better place in which to live. Unfortunately, some of the managers were motivated exclusively by external rewards and seldom spoke of "healing," "charity," or "vocation." Using a similar reward system for all managers produced rebellious, cynical subgroups and decreased motivation and productivity. No matter how hard this CEO tried, an affiliative mission whose core values were healing and caring made no impression on managers who, in philosophy and practice, would have felt right at home with a CEO named Niccolo Machiavelli.

At the time this was written, this CEO is still struggling to find a solution to the problem. Should he terminate the high-performing, business-focused managers and hire more caring replacements? Is there any hope of getting his managers to "meld into" the organization's mission and value system? Ultimately, he may have to compromise and use different forms of motivation on different managers, depending on their personal values profiles. One thing is certain: In designing any system, this CEO must always keep the mission in mind. The ship's captain does not ask the crew where the ship should go. If the crew does not want to go to the ship's destination, then they should leave the ship.

> "We must engender trust and confidence through consistency. Credibility is the key to leading others."
>
> —*Raymond A. Graeca*, CHE, *president and* CEO, *DuBois Regional Medical Center, DuBois, Pennsylvania*

Creating the Vision: Where Are You Headed?

Once you know why your organization exists and what you believe in, you can decide where you want to go. In structuring your vision, you should move through a three-step process, as described in the following paragraphs.

First, describe the direction and goals of the organization. Choose only a direction that relates to your mission and value system. This direction may involve a number of categories, including the following:

- *Social:* demographics, escalating patient expectations, changing values about work and family, growth of the elderly population, changes in ethnic compositions
- *Technological:* information systems, decision support systems, artificial intelligence, pharmaceutical advances, medical developments, preventive strategies, ethical issues, reimbursement
- *Economic:* regulation of charges, determination of services and sites, establishment of payment procedures, influence of health staffing tort reform
- *Environmental:* changes in diet, smoking, teenage pregnancy, alcohol and substance abuse, AIDS, homelessness, the uninsured, the aging
- *Staffing:* malpractice, payment limitations and variations, cost of medical education, supply and retention of nurses and allied health professionals

"The two best ways to inspire followers is first, create a values context, and second, help all staff make a connection between their behavior and the values."

—Celia Michael, PH.D., New Mexico VA Healthcare System, Albuquerque

Second, examine the implications of your vision. What does the vision mean? What is its potential impact? How might this vision influence physicians, trustees, nurses, and allied health professionals? What does it mean for your organization in terms of human resources, finance, facilities, programs and services, marketing, planning, governance, and community relations? Gauge the systemic impact of your vision on various groups within the hospital as well as on current divisions, department functions, or special constituencies. In pursuing this line of argument, ask questions such as the following:

- *Social:* How could the aging of the baby boom generation affect your approach to wellness and prevention of disease? How might an increase in AIDS cases affect your hospital?

- *Economic/public policy:* What will be the impact of changes in methods of reimbursement? How might the health system affect patient discharge, limitation of care to the severely ill, or outpatient services? Will your hospital one day be forced to close its doors?
- *Technological:* Are you able to afford new technologies? What technologies should be given priority? How much will technology reduce the cost of healthcare? How much will it increase operational costs? Given your mission and service area, what technologies will be necessary? How will reimbursement affect your purchase and use of technology?
- *Staffing:* How will the growing shortage of nurses and allied health professionals affect your organization? Will you be able to attract primary care physicians and specialists to your organization and area?

> "The more physicians are involved, the more they will understand, feel in control of their practice, and trust the leader."
>
> —*Scott Nygaard*, M.D., *chief medical officer and senior vice president of medical affairs, Affinity Health System, Menasha, Wisconsin*

Third, discuss the strategic and tactical plans needed to achieve your vision. What are the broad strategies that you plan to pursue? The following questions may be considered:

- *Technological:* Are you abreast of developments in technology as well as changing reimbursement patterns? Have you educated your public about technological developments and dilemmas?
- *Social:* Do you offer services adapted to the needs of working women, the aged, teenage mothers, those who are seriously overweight, and the drug and alcohol addicted?
- *Staffing:* How can we restructure the environment to give nurses and ancillary personnel more professional responsibilities and more opportunities to advance?

- *Economic:* Have you enhanced efficiency (in response to declining reimbursement) through innovative staffing, techniques, new purchasing methods, and the establishment of alternative sites?

EXERCISE: CREATING A VISION STATEMENT

This exercise is designed to help you articulate your vision for your department, division, or organization. A vision has several characteristics. Discuss each one separately before writing out a vision statement.

Visions are statements of destination, so they are forward looking. How far into the future are you able to look?

_____

_____

_____

Visions are conceptualizations of hopes for the future. They state what the end results should look like. Using words and phrases, describe your desired end results.

_____

_____

_____

Visions express a sense of the possible, not the probable. They are expressions of the ideal, the standard of excellence. Describe what you want to have happen (not what you think will happen) in your vision.

_____

_____

_____

Visions are unique: they set you apart from everyone else. This singularity fosters commitment. Describe how your vision would set you apart from others.

_____

_____

_____

The job of the leader is to communicate his or her vision to others and to gain their commitment to that vision. Review your previous statements and then write a vision statement in 25 words or less.

_____

_____

_____

If you feel really ambitious, try to reduce this statement to a ten-word sentence.

_____

_____

_____

REFERENCES

Atchison, T. 2003. "Exposing the Myths of Employee Satisfaction." *Healthcare Executive* 18 (3): 20–26.

Lauer, C. S., S. J. Samaha, S. L. Furry, and G. Hickman. 2002. "Straight Talk: New Approaches in Healthcare. Clinical Information Systems: Where Are We Today, Where Do We Need to Be, and How Do We Get There?" *Modern Healthcare* 32 (4): 73–76.

Nolan, K. 2003. Interview with author.

CHAPTER 8

Action:
Implementing Successful Changes

THE ASSESSMENT AND analysis are done. Strengths and weaknesses have been assessed and analyzed on the basis of desired corporate culture. Now it is time to take action. The action plan specifies what will be done, who will be responsible for its various components, how rapidly the plan will move forward, and what metrics will be used to determine progress. It is, of course, the human factors that must underpin the plan of action, including the highly important motivation, meaning, and pride.

Think of an executive who is overstressed because of the number of changes and the pace of those changes in her hospital. For years she has felt her predicament worsen and constantly recites to herself a litany of potential perils and risks. She has endured self-righteous lectures by well-intentioned friends on the human value of her work environment. But the question still remains: What can she do about inspiring followers to understand the need for change? Part of the answer rests in her ability to look inward and ask herself fundamental, albeit difficult, questions: Who am I—as a person and as a professional? What am I expected to accomplish, and will the accelerating pace of change prevent me from achieving my goals? The way she chooses to define her leadership style will determine her ability to create followers who can cope with the changes needed to succeed.

REASONABLE GOALS

To take action means that leaders must operationalize the culture by translating it in ways that create followers. What is possible? What is realistic? What will work? What resources—time, talent, energy, money—will be needed to make this action plan work? How can I engage, inspire, and align followers? In an interview for the *Journal of Healthcare Management*, Warren Bennis says, ". . . effective leaders . . . have to actually provide purpose, enable authentic relationships among their people, have a sense of hardiness themselves, and, finally, have courage to take risks—basically the capacity to act" (Johnson 1998).

If the organization is already troubled by dysfunctional individuals, the leader has several deceptively simple options available to deal with the situation. He can (1) terminate the current band of organizational cynics and find appropriate replacements, (2) introduce strategies to change their behavior, or (3) identify new strategies to inspire them to become more productive.

Typically, real action requires all three options. When to use which option is decided by the leader who again must consider the organization's culture and ask himself, What are we trying to achieve? What is our purpose? Then, he must determine which individuals will become followers and contribute constructively to achieve the mission and which are more likely to sabotage its fulfillment. The only two courses of action are to change the culture and to change the people.

Hard-core titled executives may take what looks like the easy way out and move swiftly toward termination and replacement of organizational renegades. But leaders who weather the assessment and analysis process often discover that their problems are more complex than they had anticipated and not easily resolved by eliminating people. Why? In the course of determining what inspires followers, leaders often discover that the problem is the product of weak relationships among employees, their jobs, and the organization. Most issues lie in misaligned or inappropriate systems.

For example, a healthcare executive who completes the assessment and analysis process may discover that she has 50 senior and middle managers who are more motivated by affiliation and caring than by achievement. At about the same time, the organization reaffirms that "productivity is our number one priority." Will well-meaning, good-hearted, very caring, risk-averse people be effective in this organization? Is it possible to motivate them to place less emphasis on caring and more on achievement? The answer is no. Changing goals cannot change one's motivational influences. Can their jobs be restructured to blend caring with achievement? Or should the organization do an about-face and boldly assert, "Caring is our number one priority"?

Organizations face similar pressures when external events force a change in culture. A flamboyant CEO of a Midwest community hospital put together a hard-driving management team composed of executives who were primarily motivated by recognition and money. In the wake of reduced payments and greatly increased competition, however, the organization has begun to cut back its services and staff and has redefined its mission to state, "We're going to do more with less and stress high quality and consumer satisfaction." Is it any wonder that a management group accustomed to basking in the limelight and seeing tangible rewards in its paychecks would start to feel confused, angry, and demoralized? What, then, can the CEO do? Should he try to transform his managers and persuade them to accept the wisdom of "small is beautiful"? Should he try to discover other, nontraditional ways to provide recognition and compensation? Or should he change the newly articulated mission and values? The fundamental challenge of action is to align inherent motivational drives with corporate goals. Alignment is the key to followership.

The CEO described above faces a typical crisis of executive action. Where are we going? What can we do? What is possible, realistic, and workable? How serious is our "illness"? Will antibiotics be sufficient, or is major surgery needed? In many cases, the executive concludes that the organization needs both. These executives find it tough to accept the reality that ambition and good intentions are no guarantee of success. It is impossible to have followers without alignment of personal values and corporate culture, and it is impossible to call yourself a leader if there are no followers.

To use an analogy, it would be futile to offer someone a million dollars to grow seven feet tall, because no amount of money would help the person achieve that goal. In the same way, it is useless to offer people corner offices, leased automobiles, and expense accounts if they lack the ability to fulfill your expectations. First create the ecosystem (culture) that leverages the inherent drives of the followers. This is how Kevin Nolan, of Affinity Health System (Menasha, WI); Greg Carlson, CHE, of Owensboro (KY) Mercy Health System; and Kelly Mather, of Sutter Lakeside Hospital (Lakeport, CA) transformed their cultures.

Leaders understand that the more you push in a direction counter to people's nature, the more they will rebel. Put another way, the greater the pressure to achieve the impossible, the greater the frustration (which may turn into passive or active aggression), anger, and apathy. A nurse may covertly attack the supervisor who again and again brings up the importance of the bottom line during annual evaluations. An accountant may turn corporate values into a company joke by filling every memo and report with lofty phrases and euphemisms. Others may expend their energy trying to prove that change is impossible.

Too many executives believe that they can set up expectations, introduce incentives, and communicate a positive attitude and thereby get the results they want. But the gospel of "stretch for success" is effective only when followers are aligned toward a goal consistent with their personal goals, needs, and expectations. If they feel disenfranchised and demoralized, everyone loses—especially the organization. Communicating expectations with only limited understanding of followers' needs can cause traumatic effects on people and become a form of slow-motion organizational suicide. Leaders, on the other hand, avoid empty rhetoric, and followers respond to integrity.

What exactly, then, can leaders do? First, they can align expectations so that followers see how they fit into the action plan. In the meantime, they discuss expectations with other senior executives and physicians to determine if their goals are realistic and workable. Next, they can build safety nets for followers so that they have the opportunity to take some risks, experiment with a new behavior or skill, and develop a sense of how they can best achieve their part of the action plan. At the same time, leaders must exercise patience with followers who try to change but fail the first few times. Followers can learn a great deal in "safe" failures such as pilot tests. Finally, leaders need to take followers as far as they are able to go and give them every opportunity to succeed. They accept the reality that some will not succeed and that those who do not may have to be replaced.

> "I believe that leadership and followership [are] situational. However, there are two fundamentals regardless of the situation. First, followers want to know that they are cared about and will be cared for. The second key to inspiring followers is they must believe that the leaders is competent. This is the same for the military as well as civilian healthcare."
>
> —CAPT *Anthony Sebbio*, MSC, USN, CHE

Tell a person who wants to begin a modest exercise program to get ready to run a 26-mile marathon in eight days, and she may end up hating you. Even worse, she may grow so discouraged that she will do nothing. But give that same person a specific, achievable goal such as walking for a half-hour four times a week, and she may thank you for getting her started on the road to better health. A useful mantra for this concept is "think small, move fast, evaluate, and celebrate."

Keep the goal within reach, and your followers will build a strong culture based on successful achievement of small, vision-specific tasks that they own and take pride in accomplishing.

In moving from assessment to analysis to action, leaders must identify the barriers to achieving the organization's vision. How formidable are the barriers? Can they be eliminated? Who are the followers who will be able to effect the change? What do they need to be successful? If the barrier is too great for the present staff members to surmount, the leader has the choice of changing expectations or changing people. To stand stoically by and hope things improve is folly; hope is not an effective strategy for change. Everyone will grow frustrated and angry, and the organization will falter in the process.

IDENTIFYING ESSENTIAL CHANGE ELEMENTS

Once an executive decides that his cadre of followers can fulfill the organization's mission, are prepared to accept its values, and can achieve its vision, he is ready to initiate the change process by identifying the essential change elements. Essential change elements ask this key question: To fulfill our mission in the context of our values and to achieve our vision, what do we need to change? Table 8.1 shows the ten culture change targets Affinity Health System (AHS) used to begin its transformation process.

Debbie Grogan-Wood, senior vice president of human resources, asked the staff of each area to list all the barriers to improving in these ten target areas and to describe how difficult it will be to remove each of them. As a starting point, they gave special attention to specific behaviors and policies, focusing on these questions: What behaviors and policies detract from or enhance staff performance? Which of these barriers can we eliminate, and which must we accept? This process was very helpful in creating followers who feel more empowered as managers.

Table 8.1: AHS's Ten Critical Success Areas

Statement	Baseline 2001	Target 2002
• What this system values is clear to its workers.	48%	74%
• This system has clearly defined priorities.	48%	74%
• This system is clear about what it expects from me as an employee.	62%	78%
• I take pride in being part of this system.	67%	84%
• I have a sense of loyalty to this system.	68%	85%
• I identify with this system.	53%	80%
• People are always getting extra awards and extra benefits by doing good work.	9%	54%
• I regularly receive information about the quality of my work.	32%	67%
• In this system, we hear more about what people do right than the mistakes they make.	25%	62%
• This system makes me feel like I'm an important, productive person.	30%	65%

The goal of all leadership is to produce self-managed followers. Everything in the organization should be reviewed with the aim of encouraging followers to think like responsible adults rather than like children, victims, or interchangeable parts of a machine. Consider the issue of time. If people are burdened—especially professional-level staff—with rigid time and attendance requirements, they will very likely become clock-watchers. They will perform assigned tasks and functions within the specified hours and then bolt for the door. If the goal is to stimulate people to move faster and farther than ever before, the focus should be on achieving goals. If the goal is quality and high performance and not discipline and conformity, followers must be free from the often oppressive shackles of time commitments, especially time spent in meetings.

In seeking out the essential change elements of the organization, you should scrutinize several areas: recruitment, employment and hiring, orientation, communication, recognition, rewards, compensation, incentives, re-recruitment of high performers, and termination procedures. Certain questions should be asked about each of these areas, such as, What is it about the way we hire, orient, communicate with, or reward people that stands in the way of achieving our vision? What factors can we eliminate to decrease destructive, internal competition and help our followers feel more valued and appreciated?

"Friendliness is a big factor. When I started working here I spent hours meeting with staff. I wanted them to know that they could call me Jeff and that I was always available to them. A leader must be seen first as a person."

—*Jeffrey K. Norman, executive vice president/chief operating officer, St. Vincent's Health System, Jacksonville, Florida*

In conducting this inquiry, you should take a realistic approach. For example, it is a myth that removing one bad apple or even an entire bag of apples will automatically alleviate or cure a system's problem. The absence of a negative is not a positive, although removing a negative does make a positive more likely. The problem may be so deeply embedded in the job or organization that not even wholesale firings or a major restructuring will solve it.

Although converting or otherwise transforming individuals and groups may be beyond a leader's power, organizational systems can be altered. If staff and physicians have felt oppressed, victimized, or intimidated by these systems, even minor adjustments may cause them to behave differently.

A leader inspires followers because she continually discusses the organization's essential change elements in terms of the mission, values, and vision. She reviews followers' perceptions and tries to build a commitment by addressing questions such as these: Is this the business purpose we all feel committed to? Are these the core convictions that are important to us? Is this the direction in which we want to go?

TAKING ACTION: YOUR ROLE IN THE CHANGE PROCESS

The following guidelines may help you when introducing a change process:

- Understand that there are no quick fixes when it comes to human behavior. Change takes time—sometimes months, even years. It took three years for AHS to transform itself. Exercise patience and compassion, but know when to cut losses if the situation appears hopeless.
- Remember that no follower can do everything, no matter how noble the intentions or how strong the expectations.
- Take time to document and discuss the differences between your vision of the organization and current realities. Once followers understand the gap, they will become more sensitive to what it will take to move forward.

Once the essential change elements have been established, people will be eager to move ahead. You can then ask the following series of questions:

- What is stopping us?
- What aspects of the organization must be changed?
- What aspects must be repaired or rectified?
- What aspects must be eliminated?
- What elements must be added?

Consider the example of the woman who needs to lose 50 pounds. She understands why she should lose weight and looks forward to increased energy, health, and attractiveness. She can envision herself as a more buoyant and active person with a lower cholesterol count. Her first question is important: What is it about the way I live my life that must be changed? As a start, she will have to stop eating 650-calorie blueberry muffins for breakfast and going out for pitchers of beer after work. Knowing what to stop is a good first step, but the next question is even more critical: Now that I know what must be stopped, how do I behave positively? At breakfast, she will probably substitute low-calorie cereal, fruit, and skim milk for muffins. Diet soft drinks and mineral water will become the staples of her after-work get-togethers. In addition, she will "snack-proof" her refrigerator by filling it with low-calorie foods; she will even take care not to drive by her favorite fast-food haunts.

Aside from substituting and eliminating some behaviors, she will also add new elements to her life: a half-hour, four-times-a-week exercise program; a daily 20-minute meditation session to control stress; and a regular class in pen-and-ink drawing to provide a diversion from eating.

> "All followership comes down to trust. I even have a dedicated e-mail called the 'CEO Link.' Any staff can send suggestions, ask me questions, or share a problem."
>
> —Vicki L. Romero, president and CEO, Longview Regional Medical Center, Longview, Texas

Organizations must take a similar approach. Identification of barriers that must be reduced or eliminated will produce several common themes that can then be translated into essential change elements. These elements are critical to strengthening the organization's culture.

In many cases, it is intangible factors such as trust, respect, concern, and pride that will be identified. Typically, people will make statements like these: "We want to feel better about working here," "We want to relate better to coworkers," and "We want to spend less time gossiping and bickering." As a group identifies essential change elements, it asks these two questions about each one: Is this element critical to strengthening our culture? Are we committed to changing this critical element?

GUIDELINES FOR CHANGE

Once the organization's vision has been articulated, the team can ask the following questions: What changes must be made around here? What needs to be done to make this vision come true? What barriers must be destroyed, accepted, or lowered if we are to achieve our vision and fulfill our mission? What *must* change?

Decisions on these essential change elements must be rooted in the organization's culture. If the culture is weak, a cultural enhancement process is needed. The first step here would be to refer back to the organization's baseline assessment. AHS selected the ten essential change elements listed in Table 8.1 from 200 possible elements.

In identifying essential change elements, a leader may want to take the following advice:

1. Make sure the entire team understands where the organization is headed.
2. Engage team members in a process to reach consensus on the essential change elements—what it will take for the organization to succeed, and what barriers presently exist that inhibit achievement of the vision.
3. Reach agreement on how the group will identify the essential change elements. Take the time to explain the entire process and its expected outcomes before beginning.
4. Begin with the mission statement as already developed and approved. If the group's focus wavers, remind its members of the organization's vision.
5. Reinforce the notion that all essential change elements must be seen as barriers to achievement of the vision.
6. Request that team members abide by certain guidelines such as, "everyone must contribute to the process"; "every idea, no matter how outrageous, deserves a hearing"; "there should be no challenging, criticizing, or ridiculing of ideas"; and "all ideas must be written down and reviewed."

7. Begin each essential change element statement with "We must . . . "
8. Focus on the organization, not on specific departments or individuals. For example, if someone declares, "We need to get rid of that loser in finance," turn the discussion to the types of behavior that must be eliminated or enhanced if the organization is to succeed. Always distinguish people from behaviors.
9. Limit the number of essential change elements to no more than eight and no fewer than four. Consolidate essential change elements to the minimum number required to achieve your vision.
10. Devote each essential change element to a single issue.
11. Be prepared to invest at least three hours in the entire process.

Identifying Change Elements

In developing the list of essential change elements, the leader will want to move through the accompanying five-step, 180-minute exercise with the key members of the leadership team.

Exercise: A Process for Identifying Essential Change Elements

Step One: Take 30 minutes to silently generate ideas on the following three questions:
1. What are the main issues or problems surrounding this organization?
2. What programs, services, or remedies would help us deal with these problems?
3. How can we best implement these programs or services?

Step Two: Take 45 minutes to complete a round-robin listing of ideas on a flip chart.

Step Three: Take 60 minutes to ask for clarification on each idea.

Step Four: Ask each individual to silently list and rank the ideas for 30 minutes.

Step Five: Take 15 minutes to discuss the ranking.

Some of the essential change elements generated by this exercise may be very broad; others may be very specific. They may range from "we need a better system of evaluating performance" to "we need to eliminate destructive gossip among department managers." Consider the following sample list of essential change elements:

1. We must invest in state-of-the-art information systems.
2. We must improve communications with the various segments of the public that use the hospital.
3. We must enhance the organization's self-concept and self-esteem.
4. We must document our service to the community.
5. We must create mechanisms for making ethical decisions on resource allocation.
6. We must monitor, track, and motivate our workforce.
7. We must learn to serve a diverse population.

If the essential change elements are identified by a group, they must be accepted as valid baselines on which to build improvement processes. At that point, the group will be ready for a more detailed analysis of the elements, as follows:

1. *Why should we change?* Briefly restate the reasons for change. How will the organization benefit from this change? In what ways will things improve?
2. *How should we change?* Briefly identify a broad approach for addressing each essential change element. For example,

Essential Change Element	Strategy
Track motivation of workforce	Repeat annual assessment
Support ethnic diversity	Identify people's customs and lifestyles
Improve communication	Provide education and better technology, mentors
	Communicate service
	Develop new linkages, feedback systems

3. *How will we know that we have achieved our vision?* Identify the criteria by which team members will evaluate their success. For example,

Essential Change Elements	Criteria
Track motivation	Fewer complaints, less sabotage
Support ethnic diversity	Better responses from opinion leaders
Improve communication	
Communicate service	Quicker response times
	Strong positive responses to customer satisfaction surveys

Behaviors to Address Change Elements

From the essential change elements will come a small number of specific behaviors that will in turn become the focus of performance. These behaviors can be classified according to one of the two following systems:

System 1

People: Build more management depth in professional service. Strengthen the management skills of nurses.

Systems: Develop an approach to termination that provides for successful outplacement. Connect incentive systems to achievement of the organization's vision.

Policies: Redefine leave policies to allow for management sabbaticals. Change time and attendance policies to accommodate varied work styles.

Procedures: Move the requisition of office supplies from the central supply area. Permit individual managers to make decisions concerning the use of express mail or facsimile transmittal without supervisor approval.

System 2

Rewards/Recognition: Provide service awards to employees who embody organizational values. Involve family members in more organizational events.

Achievement: Develop organizationwide systems to ensure improved quality of service.

Power: Increase the organization's visibility in the local and national media. Develop stronger relationships with legislators and business groups.

Affiliation: Offer followers a nonpunitive vehicle for discussing complaints, potential problems, and grievances. Increase involvement by community members on committees and special advisory councils.

Take care not to position essential change elements along divisional or professional lines, and avoid discussions that chronicle the faults and foibles of physicians, trustees, managers, dietitians, or any other professional group. Avoid "the negative vortex of doom"—they are the toxic workplaces described earlier in the book. Instead, keep the focus on systematic changes that will reinvigorate the entire organization.

By concentrating on a few specific essential change elements, managers can make a concerted effort to implement these behaviors throughout the organization. The essential change elements are derived from the analysis of barriers to achieving the organization's vision. The implementation of these behaviors will result in a reduction of the barriers, a strengthening of the culture, and sustainable followership.

TURNING ESSENTIAL CHANGE ELEMENTS INTO ACTION

Once the essential change elements have been identified and translated into specific behaviors, they can be implemented by leaders throughout the organization. The next step, then, is to turn once again to a consideration of the organization's mission, values, and vision. For example, if the core organizational values include justice, quality, fairness, and respect for the individual, the leader must determine whether those values are in fact addressed by the essential change elements. If not, perhaps the organization will simply spin its wheels as it attempts to change the wrong behaviors and confuse potential followers.

Moving into action demands measurable performance plans—specific events and checkpoints that detail who does what, when, where, and how. After each leader develops an individual performance plan for each behavior, she must describe how things will be different once changes have been made.

In the midst of the change process, healthcare leaders often realize the wisdom of the saying "Little things mean a lot." Suppose the essential change element is to enhance recognition, and the leaders will have achieved success when people say thank you more often. Unfortunately, many titled executives scoff at change on this seemingly basic level. "Of course, I appreciate my people," they claim. "I thank them all the time." To test the validity of this kind of assertion, one executive kept a one-day tally of his thank you behavior. Surprised at his score up to 4:00 p.m., he began to say thank you deliberately just to amass a respectable score. Although he appreciated people's contributions, saying thank you simply was not in his repertoire of behavior. On the basis of one insight, that executive now relates to colleagues and coworkers in a dramatically different way.

This titled executive's response was only one example of how his organization had to change from the top down. If that organization wanted to make the value of recognition come alive, there would be nothing more powerful, more easy, or less expensive than having that executive—and others like him—say, "Thanks a lot for your help. I really appreciate the way you took care of things for me."

For leaders, the lesson is clear. They have learned to appreciate the power of the individual. If 1,000 employees changed one thing about their behavior that would help the organization fulfill its mission and achieve its vision, 1,000 changes would occur and the positive consequences generated would be massive. Take this idea a little further: If each of those individuals changed one behavior each quarter, about 4,000 changes a year would be produced.

One of the leader's roles is to make positive, vision-focused change a routine event for all followers. To reinforce the importance of such change, people need to be asked to regularly record or note positive behaviors. They should then consider the following questions: What effect did the change have on their behavior? What was the impact of the change on others? How will the new behavior change their relationships? Most importantly, they need to share with others the ways in which they have changed. In one hospital, the leader described how he had changed his strategy for terminating an employee. In previous years, he often forced employees to resign through harassment and intimidation. Just as often, however, the employee stayed around long enough to sabotage projects and spread resentment. After practicing a simple three-step process—define, discipline, and discharge—the leader reported that he could compassionately terminate an employee, protect the culture, and avoid the pain of interpersonal conflict.

For a leader, the strategy for implementing organizational change is as follows:

- First, recommend ways for taking note of behavioral improvements. This might be as simple as a tally in a notebook or a daily entry in a work diary.
- Second, create ways for followers to share their change experiences with others. At the beginning of each major meeting, forum, retreat, or professional development program, refer back to the organization's mission, values, and vision to provide a context for any changes that may be discussed.
- Third, share personal change experiences, especially those that relate to the organization's mission, values, and vision. It takes courage for a leader to admit before a group, "I went out of my way to help a patient with a problem today. Before we started this process of looking at who we are and where we are headed, I would have blamed someone else for the problem or passed the buck. But today, I took a small part of my day to help someone who really needed it."
- Last, give followers the support they need to make changes. If this requires development of a particular skill, make sure that the appropriate program is instituted. It is futile to encourage people to be innovative if they do not have the necessary cognitive and behavioral skills.

To begin the change process, people must be challenged to share at least one thing they plan to change each week for a series of weeks. Then, people must begin the process within 24 hours of the initial meeting.

In an effective organization, everyone—from the chair of the board to the dietary services worker—has made a commitment to changing in ways that will help the organization achieve its vision. Just as the would-be dieter can make a commitment to lose four ounces a day, so can people within an organization achieve success by committing themselves to making one small change and then repeating the process over and over again.

Therein lies the difference between titled executives and leaders. In their zeal to change things as quickly as possible, titled executives often autocratically force solutions on others. Leaders, in contrast, inspire followers to solve their own problems by giving them realistic goals and the confidence and power to attain them. Becoming obsessed with detail and data, titled executives sometimes begin to act like lords of the manor. But leaders have the courage to share their continual struggle to overcome their own weaknesses. They also know that, no matter what, they will survive, and they realize that genuine power comes from empowering others, not withholding power. Leaders are the best role models for action because they display more appropriate behaviors more often.

> "Leaders hold people accountable while asking 'How can I help?' Leaders must be personal, be credible. I also believe that humor and humility are important factors that attract followers."
>
> —*Curtis Chastain*, M.D., *president, Lake Primary Care Physicians, Our Lady of the Lake Regional Medical Center, Baton Rouge, Louisiana*

Above all, leaders are willing to confront reality. Leaders welcome "brutal metrics." Unlike the fabled emperor in his "new clothes," they will never self-righteously parade through the streets while their followers cheer in blind adulation. Nor will they imitate the Queen of Hearts in *Alice in Wonderland* and rampage through the hallways screaming "Off with their heads!" at the slightest sign of deviant behavior.

Unfortunately, however, the Queen of Hearts's vindictive scenario is still practiced in too many organizations. One CEO has earned the nickname "the Terminator" because of the way she treats employees who dare to question her authority. Before meetings, managers must print their questions on blank cards and hand them to an associate who screens them lest the CEO be embarrassed by any "stupid" or "inappropriate" queries. Needless to say, few bold, innovative, or aggressive leaders stay longer than a year.

The effective leader, in contrast, creates a conflict-free environment where everyone in the organization—from the president of the medical staff to the laboratory technician—feels liberated to think and dream. An unwritten rule undergirds every action: "This is a safe place to work. I can offer criticism and suggest better ways for doing things with no fear of reprisal. No one will hurt me for being honest and direct in helping the organization fulfill its mission."

Above all, the leader must lead the change process by example. If the titled executive does not model the desired behavior, no one will. One of the most demoralizing experiences for members of an organization is to hear a CEO say, "It's your problem; you fix it." Sometimes employees are not even aware of the problem, let alone of the most appropriate solution to it.

To be effective, senior leadership must lead through modeling and be willing to share—on a highly personal level—their difficulties in grappling with change and experimenting with new behaviors. A model CEO said at a staff meeting, "I'm struggling with these economic demands. We're successful now, but I want you to know that it's not easy. I came into healthcare because I wanted to help people, and now I spend most of my time looking at financial forecasts. But I've decided to limit my financial planning to the afternoons and use my mornings for creative work. I'm going to work on human capital as hard as I work on financial capital. What do you plan to do?"

As a leader works through the change process, she must keep the focus on the barriers to achieving the organization's vision and not on day-to-day problems. If she focuses on problems, she may contract a near-fatal case of "analysis paralysis." When the focus is on barriers, there is only one issue at hand: "Here's the barrier. Are we going to reduce it, eliminate it, or accept it?"

In fact, once followers are inspired, they can deal with almost any barrier that stands in their way. Like the crew of a ship, they will never stray from their ultimate destination simply because they run into bad weather. Instead, they will decide—as a team—whether to change course or ride out the storm. Rather than fret about the fate that might befall them, they will focus on home port and their reason for going to sea in the first place.

Organizations are much the same. If senior management sets a negative example through an obsession with finances, the organization probably will never build a strong bottom line. On the other hand, if the leaders focus on mission, values, and vision, financial disaster will become almost impossible because the organization will have strong, committed, and proud followers.

The key to executive leadership in healthcare, as mentioned throughout this book, is to keep followers focused on how they fit into the organization's mission, values, and vision. Decisions are made on the basis of these elements and are then implemented. Followers will not lose their bearings because the leader will be present in person or in spirit to remind them of their goal. Even if they encounter barriers, the leader will have built enough momentum to carry them over the rough spots. When it comes to executing change, leaders are in the driver's seat. The choices they make as organizational role models will affect every person in the organization. Remember, leaders who are caring, engaging, and open will create an organization filled with followers who are committed, enthusiastic, and ready to seize opportunities.

> "The bottom line is that followers like feeling empowered—being allowed to do what they were hired to do. Staff respond to the application of common sense that is consistent with the organization's philosophy."
>
> —Martin W. Guthmiller, CEO, Orange City Health System, Orange City, Iowa

CONCLUSION: FOCUSING ON THE TARGET

By way of conclusion, let us refer back to the change process at Affinity Health System. In that case, potential followers wanted to know at the very start what their new culture would be. When they discovered that significant changes were required, they began to put up considerable resistance.

The first step in the managed change process, then, was to overcome this resistance. Because the potential followers had high affiliation scores, it was decided to group the followers into teams as part of the change strategy. An alliance among the senior leadership of the five entities was built, and this alliance was then used to support all change actions. Several ad hoc committees were also created. One was the Guiding Coalition, used to bridge the gap from old to new. The second was a rewards and recognition committee, charged with investigating new ways to find high performance. The system also created a physician advisory team that focused on the physician involvement of the new culture and identified skills that would be needed to strengthen the quality improvement process. These skills included the business of healthcare, finance for nonfinancial planners, and marketing.

The measurable, consistent improvement in all key indicators show that the AHS cultural transformation process has achieved (and continues to achieve) its human and business goals.

REFERENCE

Johnson, J. A. 1998. "Interview with Warren Bennis, Chairman, the Leadership Institute." *Journal of Healthcare Management* 43 (4): 293–96.

PART THREE

Ensuring Organizational Vitality

CHAPTER 9

Successfully Managing the Dynamics of Change

LEADERS CONTINUALLY FOCUS on what it takes to create followers within the organization's culture. In turn, effective followership makes it possible to create and sustain a strong culture. When a leader has followers, she will be able to answer yes to the following questions: Do the followers behave in ways that reflect the core values that underpin the organization? Are they committed to the direction of the organization—its vision? Do they believe in the organization's purpose—its mission?

Creating and sustaining a strong culture means that followers live the mission, values, and vision as often as possible and in as many ways as possible. It means that followers see the leader as the master storyteller and "network anchorperson" for the organization's identity, direction, and beliefs.

Another important aspect of followership is its spirit. Although often lacking a visible presence, a strong spirit is expressed by followers. Diverse personalities and types of followers may populate a given cultural landscape, but they all unite around a single leader. With strong leaders, followers' commitment and job satisfaction run high. As followers increasingly identify themselves with the organization, they create a special magic and spirit.

Even though people may be proud of their work, the workforce is never problem free. What distinguishes a strong leader is the attitude that followers take toward problems. Rather than allow problems to defeat and demoralize them, followers of strong leaders come to understand that problems are a part of life. When a problem arises, they simply say, "Here's what we're facing. How can we solve it in the context of our mission, values, and vision?" Instead of rushing to adopt the latest management trend, they faithfully turn to their context—their values and vision—to relieve the pressure of the moment.

Weak, titled executives exacerbate problems because they lack an organizational context in which to make decisions. Not having an overall focus, titled executives turn to their personal value systems—that is, their self-interest—for direction. A leader will forge diverse personal values into focused followership, thereby channeling everyone's energy toward organizational improvement. Weak titled executives give people nothing to believe in but themselves. Compelled to use their own values as a basis for making decisions, they are inclined to think, You haven't given me anything to believe in, so I'm going to make decisions that serve my own best interests.

Followers always turn to corporate values and vision when making decisions. Leaders help followers arrive at decisions in the context of a corporate value system that is larger than any individual or any group of individuals. Titled executives, in contrast, force people to think of themselves first. Without a transcendent purpose, we all default to survival.

Organizational improvement can be viewed either as an opportunity or as a source of conflict. Conflict thrives in weak cultures in which self-interest rules. Although people may appear to be arguing about how to solve a problem, their arguments usually reflect a lack of an organizational focus. Witnessing these conflicts, managers resort to traditional conflict-resolution techniques when they should be building a permanent context for organizational improvement. Improving the organization and resolving conflicts involve very different dynamics.

At some point during the evolution of a conflict, titled executives seem to make the unconscious decision to turn a chance for improvement into a conflict. For example, to address the issue of nurse recruitment and retention, a titled executive may decide to increase the nurses' pay by 15 percent, thereby seemingly solving one problem. Understandably, pharmacists, physical therapists, occupational therapists, and ancillary staff grow bitter and resentful at the special treatment accorded to nurses. They begin to think only of personal survival, both in financial terms and in terms of self-worth.

Leaders focus on the broad issue of how all of the followers deliver care and ask how everyone—not just the nurses, the professionals who deliver healthcare—can work together to deliver high-quality healthcare and how we can bring them together to increase commitment to our patients. What are nurses doing now that can be done successfully by others? What systems can be changed to improve the working conditions for all caregivers?

A leader can position a challenge in the context of an organization's vision and values. But if the titled executive is weak, he will be more inclined to examine a problem in isolation. Instead of looking at it in context, he may try to push it to the side or find someone to blame, or he may try to make a few quick-fix repairs. Leaders thrive on challenges; titled executives thrive on conflicts.

ROLE MODELING

The most powerful weapon in inspiring followers is a leader who can function as a role model. Members of the workforce—potential followers—will put more credence and faith in a leader's behavior than in speeches, memos, or the glowing message at the front of the annual report. What he does counts for much more than what he says. People *listen* to behavior.

The critical intangible factor that maintains followers is trust. Trust results from consistent, reliable, and predictable behavior on the part of leaders. Followers have faith that the leader will continually say and do the right thing for the organization. Once he says one thing and does another, that bond of trust is broken—not to be easily or quickly repaired. Trust is very hard to develop and easy to weaken, and it must be earned every day. Titles are given, but trust is earned. Once again, anyone with a CEO title is an executive. Only leaders have followers, regardless of title.

> "The leader's role is to recognize problems and opportunities and find the best people to fix and transform the organization for the good of the mission."
>
> —*Kevin Nolan, president and CEO, Affinity Health System, Menasha, Wisconsin*

A titled executive of a large hospital may talk a good line about productivity and organizational excellence, but the workforce knows that he invariably arrives each morning after 9:30 a.m., takes extended lunches, and then proceeds to scream at people for not getting things done. He pontificates about mission, spouts the latest management lingo, and has all the right executive props and accoutrements, but his words mean nothing to the workforce because he is unable to back up his rhetoric with action. His inconsistent and selfish behavior angers and offends the workforce and will continue to erode trust and reduce productivity.

SUSTAINING FOLLOWERS THROUGH SYMBOLS

Along with behavior and words, symbols and icons can take on an almost mystical significance for followers. A leader who understands the power of symbols uses the corporate logo to inspire followers from the cafeteria to the boardroom. Through slogans and mottoes, he continually reminds followers of the organization's purpose, direction, and value system.

Although words are necessary and important, symbols are also needed for followership. When people looked at the American flag after 9/11, they felt a rush of emotions because the flag expressed their deepest feelings about freedom, democracy, and justice. This phenomenon also occurs in organizations: Followers feel pride and personal satisfaction when they see a remodeled lobby, a beautiful playroom in the pediatrics department, or a new atrium in a skilled nursing care facility. As long as these physical changes are symbolic representations of organizational values, there must be alignment of symbols and beliefs.

Just as there must be a direct correlation between words and behavior, so there must be a direct correlation between symbols and behavior. Although mission, values, and vision are the basic ingredients of culture, trust is the glue that holds it all together. Therefore, if people note a discrepancy between the organization's symbols and icons and its behavior, the glue weakens and the culture fractures. For example, although the United States contains many diverse cultures that sometimes resemble countries within a country, it is bound together by its ability to solve problems through the rule of law. Trust breaks down when white-collar criminals are acquitted and go free. However, every time the rule of law triumphs, the system is vindicated and the bonds of trust between the people and the government are strengthened. Once trust is lost in an organization's leadership or in a nation's government, people tend to regress to selfish, turf-protecting behavior. The more distrust that exists, the more people revert to their personal value systems to make decisions and the more they resist anyone who tries to interfere with or even question their value systems. The dynamics of trust are especially true for physicians (Atchison and Bujak 2002).

How, then, is followership sustained by way of symbols? If a leader is strong, the most powerful symbolism is how she communicates the mission, values, and vision of the organization.

Her behavior must be consistent, accurate, and immediate. She does not allow wounds to fester and emotions to run over. Instead, she tackles problems immediately, clarifies their meaning, and helps people work toward solutions by building a context that is consistent with the organization's mission, values, and vision. Her daily behavior symbolized those traits that attract followers.

MANAGING CHANGE

Change is the only constant in life. There is no way to escape it. Moreover, the rate of change will, most likely, continue to accelerate in unpredictable ways. Despite these realities, many titled healthcare executives choose to deny the dynamics of change, cloaking themselves in dangerous myths that offer little more than temporary relief from reality. Consider the popularity of the following beliefs:

Myth 1: Change just happens; it can't be managed. Typical reactions include, "What happens, happens. There's nothing we can do about it"; "Let's wait and see what happens. We don't know what's going to happen until it happens, so let's not worry about it"; "What will be, will be."

Myth 2: Change can be prevented or postponed through good intentions and hard work. Standard responses are, "Things always turn out for the best"; "It will all work out"; "Let's just continue doing what we've always done"; "If it's worked for this long, it ought to keep on working"; "What was good enough for us five years ago is good enough today."

Myth 3: Change is uniform. "It's going to turn this country upside down"; "If it happened to them, it could happen to us"; "Everyone will be hurt—there is nothing we can do!"

You will not hear leaders echoing these popular myths. Leaders take a broad view of the environment and then act boldly to anticipate, manage, and direct change. Leaders follow the dictum, "You cannot predict the future, but you can prepare for it."

Likewise, the character of the healthcare industry demands that organizations have infrastructures that can absorb the shocks that will inevitably hit them. Several years ago, the head of a national health maintenance organization was on the cover of an industry news magazine as the poster child for good cost management. Shortly thereafter, the company went into bankruptcy. No matter how dazzling is a business success story or how meteoric is someone's rise to prominence, everyone is vulnerable to change.

Developing effective responses to change requires, however, that a leader understand three basic types of change: developmental change, traumatic change, and managed change.

> "All 'gods' have clay feet. Idolatry and leadership do not mix well. Seek the ideal; be grounded in reality."
>
> —Wayne Lerner, DR.P.H., FACHE, president and CEO, Rehabilitation Institute of Chicago

Developmental Change

Developmental change is inevitable in healthcare organizations. The ongoing cycle of seasons produces physical changes in the environment, and the same analogy holds true for people's bodies. No matter how well people take care of themselves, their bodies will change. To a certain extent, everyone experiences wrinkling of the skin or loss of hair. Although one can postpone, soften, or control these changes, one can never stop or reverse them. Sooner or later, aging, like winter, will happen.

The same is true of change in organizations. The x-ray was replaced by magnetic resonance imaging, which was in turn replaced by positron emission tomography. As long as resources are available for research and development, technology will expand and grow whether one chooses to invest aggressively in capital equipment, postpone purchases, or orchestrate joint ventures with other organizations.

In the same way, we can be confident that there will be continued change in legislation and regulation. In recent years, the majority of developmental changes in the healthcare industry resulted from economic pressures. While it is impossible to predict the future, we can be fairly sure that no bureaucrat, with a single flourish of a magic wand, will return healthcare to the languor of cost-based reimbursement. It is likely that the healthcare industry will see increased developmental change in areas such as managed care, availability of manpower, and consumer choice.

Following are some strategies that leaders can use in dealing with developmental change:

Create a sense of excitement about the change. Discuss the change in terms of the benefits and advantages it will offer to various sectors of the organization and to the community. If possible, show that the perceived disadvantages or problems will simply be minor, routine occurrences in the change process.

Build confidence. Help followers focus on their strengths and resources. Tell stories about how other followers successfully overcame problems and crises in the past.

Celebrate small victories and achievements. As the change progresses, share new developments with all followers in the workforce. Describe to them how each of their steps is contributing to achievement of the organization's vision.

Constantly clarify roles for followers in the context of the agreed-upon outcome. Be prepared to say to them, This is your role in ensuring the success of this new program or service.

Be patient. Give followers an opportunity to internalize the change. People need time to understand that, although they may wish to do their jobs in the same way, advantages will become apparent from the new opportunities that change will inevitably bring.

Provide forums in which followers can share issues and ask questions. Do not rely on impersonal "happiness" surveys and complaint-driven suggestion boxes. Instead, create one-on-one sessions between executives and staff members or, at a minimum, sponsor small-group sessions. Followers often need reassurance on issues as simple as, Will my work space look the same? Will I be working with the same people? How will my job change? Will I still be doing the same types of projects? Work with them to create a positive vision of how they fit into the end result.

Leaders work with followers to evaluate the implications of change for the entire organization, assessing its tangible and intangible impact on each unit and subunit of the organization and even on specific individuals. Then together they take steps to address specific problems.

Leaders exercise vigilance. They try to anticipate how changes may affect each followership unit. When changes are in the offing, they focus everyone's attention on the barriers between the present state of the organization and the vision.

Traumatic Change

Changes of this kind are typically viewed as more negative than developmental changes. The man who must cope with the developmental change of hair loss may also experience the trauma of a sports injury that leaves him bedridden for two weeks. Traumatic change can hit healthcare organizations in much the same way. Consider the following examples:

- A medical group leaves.
- The top admitter has a heart attack and dies.
- Three of the organization's top executives go to work for competitors.
- The board decides to terminate the CEO.
- A factory in the community closes, and 3,000 families of childbearing age move out.

Changes such as these can traumatize an organization, significantly affecting its ability to deliver service. On the opposite end of the spectrum, consider the following changes:

- A new factory relocates to a nearby community and brings in 3,000 new families.
- A direct mail promotion of a new weight-management program attracts 500 people who want to sign up for a complementary orientation.
- The organization receives a $5 million grant to study the effects of home visitation on the length of hospital stay.

Although positive, these changes may also generate stress and physical disruption. Traumatic change always causes people to grow possessive of their territory, space, and roles. Even a change for the better may at first produce anxiety, frustration, and confusion. Leaders inspire followers.

When an organization is hit with traumatic change, there may not be time to engage, align, and build confidence. In contrast to developmental change, traumatic change is far more likely to produce strong emotions: The most common response is fear that borders on paranoia and anger that can easily escalate into rage. Productivity can plummet as followership weakens and staff try to protect themselves from further injury and pain. In a traumatic situation, a leader needs to respond quickly. In fact, this is one of the few times when acting unilaterally may be justified. Instead of waiting for alignment to build, the leader needs to take dramatic, immediate action. People must be brought together to discuss their fears and candidly confront reality. A leader maintains followers in this way: "I realize we have a significant problem here, but together we can save this organization and everything it means to the community. We are going to focus on some specific outcomes, and while I may not have time to work with everyone, I will work with as many people as needed to make this happen."

The key difference between traumatic change and developmental change is the intensity of emotion involved and the speed with which leaders must move to defuse or redirect destructive emotions. In developmental change, a leader can rely on systematic team building; in the case of traumatic change, however, she needs to galvanize her followers by first acknowledging the problem and then outlining a strategy in which everyone can play a part. Once again, context is the key.

Following are several strategies for grappling with traumatic change:

- Recognize that communication is not a one-time event. Offer frequent progress reports and updates. No leader has ever been criticized for "overcommunicating."
- Outline the next steps that must be taken. Let all followers know when additional information will be forthcoming, as well as the specific actions that the organization plans to take and how employees fit (or do not fit) into the plan.
- Stress positive outcomes. Let followers know that the organization will survive because "we're a team."
- Make followers feel valued. Stress their indispensable role in seeing the organization through the crisis.

Of course, employing these strategies is no guarantee of success. Some followers will always blame the leader for the organization's problems. But at least they will give him some credit for acknowledging the crisis, setting the record straight, and taking steps to turn the situation around.

Another role of the leader is to short-circuit any attempts to apportion blame for the trauma. In a crisis, one invariably hears comments such as the following: "The doctors don't admit enough patients here"; "Physical therapy isn't out there recruiting more rehab patients"; "Accounting doesn't go after outstanding bills"; "The CEO is always at meetings—she doesn't care about us."

As long as failure is another person's responsibility, members of the workforce can continue to feel absolved from all blame. There can be no followership because everyone feels like the victim. Hence, the leader must persuade the followers to focus on the problem, not on one another's shortcomings: "It really doesn't matter whose fault it is. This organization is in serious trouble and unless we take action—and 'we' includes everyone from physicians to accounting clerks to dietary services workers—we may not be here in another six months. Our choice is clear: do we spend the next six months figuring out who or what is at fault, or do we pull together to save this organization? It's your choice."

It takes courage to deliver such an ultimatum. It is easy to lead during growth periods. It is very difficult to lead during times of shrinking resources. People who have shaped their identity by chronically blaming others may even look on such a leader as a traitor to the organization. But until people become followers and accept their role in solving the organization's problems, there will be little hope for that organization. Staff members must accept that their choices when facing traumatic change are to lead, follow, or get out of the way. Complaining is *not* an option.

> "Corporate culture is one of the most important ingredients in our ability to fulfill our mission. We need to be clear about what behaviors should be rewarded and what behaviors should not be rewarded."
>
> —Laurence M. Merlis, FACHE, president and CEO, Greater Baltimore Medical Center, Baltimore, Maryland

In a number of successful turnarounds in the past ten years, leaders were apparently able to perform a kind of organizational *jujitsu*; that is, they used the negative energy of the workforce to increase followership. But this is a tricky and dangerous feat. The safer, more appropriate role of the leader is to neutralize destructive behavior and to create a context in which followers are inspired to save the organization. More specifically, in addressing traumatic change, a leader's role is to give the followers permission to risk short-term failure to achieve long-term success.

Managed Change

The third kind of change is managed change. Developmental and traumatic change "fix" the past, whereas managed change anticipates the future. Leaders draw on the strength and expertise of the followers to plan for and orchestrate change by focusing on the vision. For example, turning a sleepy 200-bed community hospital into a major referral center requires a clear vision and managed change. It might mean establishing various links with the nearby university medical center. The hospital, for example, might serve as a conduit for the medical center's open-heart cases. Certainly, there would have to be major changes in how the hospital conducts its business and how the workforce perceives itself.

Managed change starts with understanding the endgame—the desired outcome. What is the organization's vision? How will the organization know when it has been successful? Articulating the desired outcome is a way of answering the questions, Where am I now, and where do I want to be? For example, if a hospital wants to increase its market share in the cardiology service line by 3 percent a year for the next five years, it first needs to determine, Where are we now? If its market share is increasing at a rate of 1 percent per year and the hospital wants to increase that rate by another two percentage points per year for five years, the next issue is to develop a strategy to accomplish this change.

Managed change is a planned process backed by a leader's ability to inspire followers to answer the appropriate questions about tangibles and intangibles: What is our business? Where are our best opportunities? In what direction do we want to go? What kind of staff do we need to execute the plan? Most importantly, how do we continue to inspire each other so that we will commit ourselves to achieving the goal? The keys to managed change are, first, the selection of the right team and, second, the creation of the shared dream—the inspirational, directional, and measurable vision.

Many titled executives forget that change is accomplished by individuals and is therefore a highly personal experience. For example, a titled executive will not effect much change with an announcement at an all-staff meeting, such as, "We're changing our market position; I expect all of you to fall in line." Managed change is not achieved by edict. Even in relatively homogeneous groups, members will have widely varying perceptions about what is important and what should or should not be changed. In the same way, although a leader can produce short-term change through the use of threats and force, he will never achieve core behavioral change that way. Simply stated, *one can change behavior only by changing people's minds and aligning their heart and soul to the desired goal.*

STRATEGIES FOR MANAGING ALL TYPES OF CHANGE

Change within an organization must be handled in the same way as change within a family. When a family faces a change in economic status, an accident, or a residential move, for example, an adult leader usually emerges to assure the other family members that everything will be fine. The mother or father, or sometimes even an older sibling, will point to the benefits of the change and urge everyone to pull together to make things better than ever.

The same is true of organizations. If a healthcare organization is located in a 60-year-old building that must be torn down and replaced with a more modern facility, employees may respond with comments such as, "It's not going to be the same"; "Why are they spending money on bricks when they could be spending money on us?"; "What's wrong with the old building?"; "We're losing our history and traditions."

The leader of that organization must carefully explain the benefits of the change to all followers. Most importantly, followers need to know that they will be able to carry out the organization's legacy for quality patient care with even greater energy and commitment in the new building. When the perception is altered from traumatic to developmental, change becomes more acceptable.

In the case of a developmental change, a leader can work systematically to mobilize the followers behind an idea. For example, when preparing to build a replacement facility, merge with another organization, or diversify into services for the elderly, the leader must develop specialized, values-based communication vehicles that align followers' interests with the changes. All opportunities must be put in place to engage the followers in the change. Followers will "own" the change by then turning developmental change into managed change.

Both as individuals and as members of the organization, people need to know that a potential change matches their personal work values and will be worthwhile and valuable. Some of the most common questions staff ask are, Do I have a role in the change process? Will I be important to its success? What am I expected to do? What happens if I fail? The role of the leader is to help potential followers know, Here's how you fit into our plans; this is what the vision means for you. For example, the obstetrics nurse who is fearful of the organization's new venture into cardiology needs to hear that the high-risk cardiology unit will focus on congenital heart problems in children. In offering that observation, the leader may not have communicated any new evidence or data to that nurse or her colleagues, other than the fact that they are critical in fulfilling the organization's vision. However, that is the most important communication of all.

> "Leaders need to look inward before looking outward. A daily dialogue with yourself will help you decide if you are doing all you can to move the organization forward. When you answer unequivocally, yes, then seek that same response in others."
>
> —*Matthew Lambert*, M.D., *FACHE, senior vice president, clinical operations, Elmhurst Memorial Healthcare, Elmhurst, Illinois*

When managing change, a leader keeps in mind that every follower is profoundly different. To effectively manage the change process, a leader needs to recognize respect and appreciate these differences.

In almost every situation other than those involving traumatic change, one needs to give followers an opportunity to align to the situation. Followers differ in their ability to process information. Some deal easily with complex ideas, while others require homespun examples, metaphors, and extended explanations. Leaders work with followers one on one, adapting the idea to the person rather than the other way around. The more a leader works with followers in developing a strong culture, the more she will come to appreciate how unique people are. Understanding and accepting their uniqueness are among the first steps in managing change. To change the behavior of those followers essential to managing change, a leader must first understand that not all human beings are equally bright, have equal or equivalent experiences, or are equally motivated. Consider a glass and a bucket both filled with water. When both are 100 percent full, one still has more capacity than the other.

In fulfilling her role, a leader must direct the motivation of the followers and move them through the process of assessment, analysis, and action. Her context for all change is a strong culture characterized by shared values, trust, and organizational commitment. If she wants to make her culture even stronger, however, she needs another skill: The ability to create strong work teams held together by trust—teams that can sustain change management in the context of the organization's mission, values, and vision without direct leadership interventions.

TEAMS AND TEAM BUILDING

I define leadership this way: A leader has followers who achieve a vision by building teams to manage change. Teamwork is a key element in sustaining followership.

Teams are used most effectively in developing new products or services, improving quality, evaluating and implementing new technology, problem solving, and quickening the decision-making process. However, Tom Peters (1987, 364), in his classic book *Thriving on Chaos: Handbook for a Management Revolution*, suggests that "the power of teams is so great that it is often wise to violate apparent common sense and force a team structure on almost everything." What are the major characteristics of teams? Whether one talks about sports teams or work teams, they have several attributes in common.

- Teams have a goal.
- Teams know the rules of the game.
- Teams know how to keep score.
- Team members understand their interdependent role in achieving the outcomes.

People are usually hired by an organization because they have the right combination of technical competence, skill, and experience. Unless they understand their role or the goal of the team, however, they cannot contribute to the team's success and may, in fact, become hindrances.

For example, John sold his skills as a public affairs specialist with Washington connections to a budding healthcare consulting firm, but he lasted only six months in his newly created vice presidential position because he never came to understand the rules of the consulting game. He failed to learn that being an entrepreneur was not compatible with long lunches, personal phone calls, and a laissez-faire attitude toward new business development. Although he was employed by an entrepreneurial company, he continued to operate by the rules of a government agency. Teams must be aligned in values and behavior.

A leader considering organizational team building needs to ask many of the same questions that a new coach or manager would ask.

- Who is on the team?
- What skills do they have?
- What game are they playing? Or what game do they think they are playing?
- What are the rules of this game, and is the team playing according to these rules?

- How does one keep score and ultimately win this game?
- How do we reward and recognize teamwork?
- What are the roles of the individual players? How can they support each other?

In a healthcare organization, an executive might ask the following questions:

- What is our target—our vision?
- How will everyone work together to reach our vision?
- What are the roles of the members of this team and of the team leader?
- How do we celebrate achievement?

Playing a game involves the risk of losing, and losing often has a more disruptive effect on people in organizations than on athletes, who are used to competing day after day. When people in organizations realize that they are unable to score enough "hits" and "runs," they may refuse to deal with the situation realistically. In such situations, both a coach and a leader need to keep followers focused on winning the game. Having someone go up to the batter's box and do ballet positions would be interesting, to say the least, but irrelevant to winning the baseball game. The same is true of the batter who chooses—just for fun—to run from third base to second base to first base. It would be intriguing, but unrelated to the task at hand. Focus on achievement—winning the game.

A leader needs to keep his followers focused, resisting the human temptation to offer interesting but irrelevant targets. For example, people may refuse to focus on solutions by denying that a problem even exists or by taking refuge in nostalgia. Typically, they will discuss what should be rather than what is. This is called *retrovisioning* and is characterized by such toxic statements as "We should have," "We would have," or "We could have." These statements place focus in the wrong (negative) direction. A leader will respond along these lines: "Yes, maybe we shouldn't have this problem, but we do. Short of divine intervention, nothing is going to change that. We need to accept that we may not be responsible for this problem but we are responsible for the solution."

The most challenging aspect of team building is role clarification. Team leaders must explain the rules of the game and clarify individual roles so that team members will understand what is expected of them and how their interdependent participation will contribute to success. Team members must also be engaged in developing strategies and tactics. This is what will build commitment to the team's goal. If the strategy is to provide better bedside care by using care providers other than registered nurses, the team leader must make sure that physicians and nurses have a say in deciding how this can be accomplished without decreasing the quality of care. In summary, the role of a team leader is to help followers understand their roles and functions on the team and give them enough focus and direction to keep participating.

An effective leader will use similar methods to mobilize the medical staff. They engage the physicians as partners to define the game, outline the rules, and figure out how everyone can become an effective team member. The greatest contribution a physician leader makes is to align the interest of the physicians to the notion that they can succeed as the organization succeeds.

> "To learn you must be vulnerable, to acknowledge that your current state of knowing is either incomplete or inaccurate. Never stop being curious; invest in diversity. Be a good listener."
>
> —*Joseph S. Bujak*, M.D., *vice president of medical affairs, Kootenai Medical Center, Coeur d'Alene, Idaho*

CONCLUSION

On the playing field or within organizations, leaders inspire followers to fulfill their roles. If players make a mistake, they may hear about it, but they also know that they can take risks and even fail because they have the confidence and support of the coach. The effective leader may chew a player out with the ear-rattling intensity of a Bobby Knight, but his last words to that player are, "All right, now let's get back out there and try it again."

It is the presence and power of the team leader that gives team followers incentive and a sense of commitment to the other players. They will rarely, if ever, let other players down. The effective coach or leader makes them feel as one: "This is a team. We play together. We win together and we lose together."

Like a good coach, the effective leader can also acknowledge personal strengths and limitations. Just as there is no way that a conductor can play all the instruments in an orchestra, so no coach could—or would want to—play all the positions on a team. Like the successful coach or celebrated conductor, the effective healthcare leader knows how to achieve the organization's vision by helping each follower to perform at his or her peak for the sake of the team.

Under the tutelage of an effective coach and leader, the superstar will excel. A truly great basketball player understands the importance of scoring fewer points and winning the game over breaking scoring records and losing the game. Contrast that with the self-indulgent player who declares, "What the rest of the team does is their own business. I'm here to score. That's how I make my money." Much to the detriment of the team, this egocentric player interprets victory and defeat from a highly selfish point of view. If the team wins, it is because he excelled; if it loses, it is because he did not get the ball enough. The effective coach or leader will know how to manage these people—by getting rid of them; neutralizing them; or giving them enough, but not too much, rope. If tensions run high, the leader or coach will control the attitude of the players through discipline. He will lift the players high above petty gripes and egotism with the words, "I don't care what you think of each other; you will play this game our way or you will not be on this team." The lessons of sports metaphors about superstars are most useful with physicians, especially subspecialists.

The role of the effective leader or coach is to select the right people, inspire and support them as well as create a spirit that binds them together with others for the achievement of the vision. A healthcare leader's responsibilities to teams include the following:

1. Develop an inspiring vision and then foster team commitment to it.
2. Create a listening environment.
3. Recognize and reward teamwork among subordinates and others who helped the team under the leader's jurisdiction.
4. Implement team projects.
5. Recruit qualified people who are enthusiastic about team participation.
6. Ensure that all professional development necessary for members of a team to function successfully is made available to them.
7. Ensure that support systems are in place.
8. Promote and encourage change, innovation, and risk taking.
9. Communicate the results of team efforts across the organization.
10. Remind players that they will either win as a team or lose as a team.
11. Build a strong team and then give its members credit for their efforts.
12. Celebrate *all* successes.

Executives must always remember that they are leaders only if they have followers. Without committed followers, a leader does not exist.

REFERENCES

Atchison, T., and J. Bujak. 2002. *Leading Transformational Change: The Physician-Executive Partnership*. Chicago: Health Administration Press.

Peters, T. 1987. *Thriving on Chaos: Handbook for a Management Revolution*. New York: HarperCollins.

CHAPTER 10

Putting It All Together: Discovering Your Followership Quotient

FOLLOWERSHIP IS THE single defining factor for leadership. Thousands of books and articles have been written about leadership, but regardless of how these texts describe effective leadership, the central question remains the same: Is anyone following you? (Atchison 1990). This book has focused on the needs, wants, hopes, and desires of potential followers. The academic and field research states that the degree to which you are able to create a workplace environment in which these followership factors are realized defines your leadership potential. For example, Margaret Wheatley's (1999) book *Leadership and the New Science* presents some provocative ideas about the "invisible" drivers of organizational performance. *Winning the Talent War,* by Carson F. Dye (2002), FACHE, shares some practical notions on the importance of aligning people and the work environment.

Viewed a different way—that is, from the employees' position —your ability to meet their needs and expectations equals your *followership quotient* (FQ). A followership quotient is simply a measure of one's ability to present a cluster of behaviors that result in a positive workplace environment in which followers thrive.

FOLLOWERSHIP QUOTIENT

Twenty-one variables comprise the FQ. This chapter presents these factors and explains how to calculate your personal FQ. Figure 10.1 shows the 21 factors and the specific domain in which they lie.

Seven developmental domains are necessary for high-performing organizations. Each domain has three elements, resulting in 21 total variables. All 21 elements need to be measured and managed. The sections that follow discuss each domain and its elements.

Domain 1: Leaders' Traits

The first domain is where most leadership texts focus. They provide information about the traits that successful leaders display. The assumption is that if you can imitate these traits, you will be a successful leader. This assumption about successful leadership traits is true to a certain degree. However, these traits must be viewed as the beginning of a chain of dependent variables that create followers who provide great healthcare services to the community. When several books and articles about leadership are analyzed for common themes, most of the information can be subclassified into three areas: intelligence, energy, and discipline.

Leadership *intelligence* is the first trait in this domain. The intelligence that inspires followers is unrelated to academic credentials. The intelligence needed to earn an academic degree is not related to the type of intelligence needed to attract followers. (In fact, some may suggest that the linear thinking needed for academic success is a barrier to the innovative thinking required of leaders.) The intelligence that attracts followers are interpersonal skills, the ability to cope quickly, and the ability to synthesize diverse opinions into creative solutions (Atchison and Bujak 2002). A unique subset of this type of intelligence is some-

Figure 10.1: Seven Developmental Domains for High-Performing Organizations

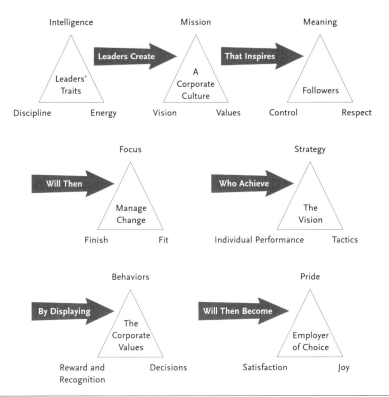

what paradoxical: This subset is a blend of courage and humility. Followers are attracted to the creative leaders who sincerely believe that the leaders are simply the conduit for the collective wisdom of their followers. Too often, the highly credentialed titled executive is viewed as arrogant because of his inability to be humble and his lack of courage, which results from an inability to focus on the contributions of others. These executives reinforce their belief in themselves by reminding themselves and others about their academic and honorific titles. They do not define themselves by the number of followers but by the number of degrees earned. Again, this is not the type of intelligence that inspires followers.

The second trait of the first domain is *energy*. Senior executives, managers, and supervisors have many demands on their time. In today's healthcare world everything seems to require attention STAT! However, the research and case studies discussed in this book suggest strongly that those in a position of power who have the greatest number of followers are the ones who spend the most time dealing with the followers' concerns. Followership seems to increase in direct proportion to the amount of perceived visibility of the leader. Recall that of all the intangibles, trust is the keystone. Furthermore, trust develops over time as a direct function of the frequency of meaningful interactions. It is impossible to trust someone you have never met or whom you only meet in a crisis mode. No one will follow someone they do not trust.

"Followers are created in an environment where their values and expectations are considered. Where they trust the leader. And where difficult issues are confronted with empathy and courage."

—*Mary Dowling, Medical Center director, VA Medical Center, Albuquerque, New Mexico*

A major part of the FQ measure is simply this: How much time is spent with those whom you wish to inspire. Do you make rounds every day, twice a day? Are your conversations with staff about meeting their needs and expectations, or is it a time to defend the status quo or worse yet to find fault? Of course, time management and priority setting are important in the trust-building process, but the fact is that those with the highest FQ *just do more* than those with low (or negative) FQs. Followers are attracted to those with high energy.

The third trait that leaders possess is *discipline*. While this characteristic is important to inspire followers in any work environment, it is especially important in today's healthcare industry, given the recent attacks on its mission. The essence of all delivery systems is to help the well and cure the sick in a way that by definition requires discipline to balance revenue and caring. The focus of last 25 years has been placed with increasing importance on the tangible, business (especially financial) issues. Too often, titled executives' emphasis on the tangibles is viewed by staff as their only discipline, resulting in common statements from staff such as "They (i.e., titled executives) care more about the budget than quality care" or "They see me only as an economic unit."

Behaviorally, followers want to see in their leaders a discipline to listen with intent to understand. Leaders seem to have a four-part discipline for effective listening: (1) attend to what is being said, (2) ask clarifying questions, (3) make a decision, and (4) determine whether the decision meets the follower's expectations (and, if it does not, why the decision was made). The executive's communication style determines whether the staff will follow. An in-depth treatment of the importance of discipline can be found in Collins's (2001) book *Good to Great: Why Some Companies Make the Leap . . . and Others Don't.*

Domain 2: A Corporate Culture

Followers are attracted to executives who possess intelligence, energy, and discipline. The first responsibility of the leader with these traits is to create a work environment, ecosystem, or corporate culture that encourages followers. This is developed through the three factors of this domain: *mission, values,* and *vision.* Corporate cultures are the way organizations behave. They are the organization's personality (Atchison 2002), and, just like in human beings, it is a very good idea to have only one personality. Healthcare organizations run by titled executives have multiple personalities, or subcultures. There is the nurse culture, and within this culture there is the surgical nurse culture and the medical nurse culture, the day shift and night shift, RN and LPN, senior and young—they all have their way of behaving. In addition, of course, there are the many physician subcultures. In fact, in a healthcare organization in which the titled executive has failed to inspire followers, there is approximately one subculture per work unit.

Corporate culture is easy to define and very difficult to create and sustain. By definition, a strong culture means that all staff units behave in a predictable way as defined by the core values. Southwest Airlines, Wal-Mart, Ritz-Carlton, and the Disney theme parks are non-healthcare entities that are used often to describe how strong cultures are manifest. The fundamental question to answer is, To what degree are our core values the main decision rule for everything we do? Consider whether the first paragraph of Lencioni's (2002, 5) article "Make Your Values Mean Something" hit home? Lencioni asks you to

> Take a look at this list of corporate values: Communication. Respect. Integrity. Excellence. They sound pretty good, don't they? Maybe they even resemble your own company's values, the ones you spent so much time writing, debating, and revising. If so you should be very nervous. These are the corporate values of Enron. . . ."

As mentioned throughout this book, corporate culture has three elements: mission, values, and vision. The mission statement addresses the question of why you exist; the set of core values answers the question of what beliefs drive decisions and underpin behavior; and the vision statement indicates where we are going and how we know we have arrived. Employees of a healthcare organization with a strong corporate culture will all be able to state, in what might be compared to the "30-second commercial," here's what we do, here's why we do it, and here's where we will be in three to five years. Because they are following someone they trust, they will also be able to tell you, "Here's how I contribute to our success." This last insight results from the element in the next domain triangle.

Domain 3: Followership

This book has tried to describe the dynamics of followership. Followership's placement in the third slot of the seven triangles needed for success shows the context in which followers exist. Without the leader possessing the right characteristics and the creation of a strong corporate culture (i.e., workplace environment/the workers' ecosystem), followers will not emerge. Followers do not happen because employees are required to attend an orientation session or one-size-fits-all management development program on customer satisfaction. They are not the consequence of a new strategic plan. And no followership has ever been sustained because you implement a new employee recognition program. The three factors that produce followers in a strong corporate culture led by inspiring leaders (i.e., the three factors of this domain) are *meaning, respect,* and *control.*

Followers find meaning in their work. All humans pay attention to those things that are important to us. The notion that employees need to be motivated is one of the most pervasive (and most toxic) myths espoused by titled executives. All human beings are 100 percent motivated 100 percent of the time to do that which has the most meaning. When the claim is made that the staff is not motivated, what is really being said is that their work has no intrinsic worth. When work has no intrinsic, intangible meaning, it must be made important by using extrinsic, tangible incentives such as money. In fact, there is an inverse relationship between intrinsic worth and the need for money as an incentive. Do you get paid to practice the religion of your choice? How much pay do you receive to raise your children? Do you get paid to travel on vacation, or do you pay others? Money is necessary to the degree that work has no meaning. An often-quoted notion reflects this relationship: "Find a job that you love, and you will never work another day in your life."

Followers thrive under leaders who create a strong culture in which they can find meaning in their work. Ask the staff what parts of their job are the most meaningful and least meaningful. After these elements are classified, ask the same staff how much time they spend on the most and least meaningful elements. A useful guideline is that when staff spend at least 80 percent on the most meaningful tasks, organizational performance, personal pride, and job satisfaction will be maximized; when less than 50 percent of the time is spent on meaningful work, performance pride, productivity, and satisfaction will be suboptimal. One of the key indicators of whether labor action will be successful is the percentage of the time staff spend on meaningful work.

The second need that followers have is for respect. For 20 years, I have been interviewing healthcare professionals in organizations contaminated with various amounts of behavioral toxins in the workplace. The main theme that emerged from thousands of these interviews is a feeling that "there is no respect for my contribution." This feeling pervades all levels and all specialties, including physicians. The irony is that most healthcare organizations profess a core value of respect. The data suggest that there is far more rhetoric about respect than actual behaviors that are perceived as respectful. Of all of the 21 factors of the FQ, respect (on the surface) seems to be the easiest to manifest, and it is the one that would result in the greatest benefit to followers. Follow these two rules to increase the amount of respect you afford your employees: (1) The rule of common sense and (2) the golden rule. Does the way I'm treating others make sense? and Would I like to be treated this way? These are two very simple rules, yet we find that respect is still an elusive feeling in most healthcare workers. Why? Is it because there are too many titled executives and too few leaders? One can only speculate about why we talk about and promote respect as a core value but the workers feel so disrespected.

> "Healthcare is a wonderful career, and the people who enter it have much to give. Only strong leadership can unlock that potential and allow creativity to flourish."
>
> —Matthew Lambert, M.D., FACHE, senior vice president, clinical operations, Elmhurst Memorial Healthcare, Elmhurst, Illinois

The third necessary for followership is control. Followers resist change when they do not understand, do not want, and/or *do not control.* Figure 10.2 shows the continuum of change.

Figure 10.2: The Easy-to-Hard Continuum

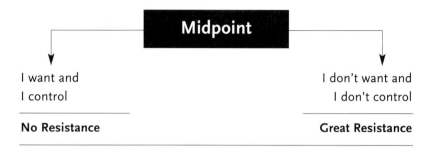

Change is not hard and not resisted when those involved understand the reasons for changing—I want the change and I control the process. Resistance increases to the degree that these factors are not present.

Employees will follow an executive who creates a workplace environment in which they feel in control of the decisions that most affect them. Control is one of the most important aspects of power. Humans must believe that they have control over their work to feel power. The power that comes from controlling the decisions that personally affect the follower is a healthy power, unlike the power that comes from passive aggressive or active aggressive behaviors to gain control, which is very toxic in health-care organizations. A simple two-question survey can identify the degree to which staff feels in control of their work: (1) What parts of your job do you control? (2)What parts of your job are controlled by others? The answers are very diagnostic, especially with physicians and nurses.

Domain 4: Managing Change

Followers who find work meaningful in a strong culture with inspirational leaders at the helm are ready to manage change. The need to change, cope, adapt, and accommodate are universal constants. The unknowns about change are the type, pace, and magnitude of the change required to survive and grow. Change is not hard to ignite. There are several techniques to launch a change process, including the following:

- creating an emergency; also known as the "burning platform"
- finding a common enemy
- creating a "burning the boats" fear of loss; that is, there is no turning back
- engineering the Hawthorne effect
- making a scheduled or unscheduled change in staffing
- experiencing an unanticipated increase in volume or complexity
- doing anything that breaks the limits of the organization's homeostasis

Trauma will always provide the incentive to change. However, trauma-driven change methodologies take a big emotional toll on the organization, and, most importantly, trauma-driven changes are *not* sustainable. Leaders understand that positive organizational change can be sustained when followers are engaged and understand the context for the change. The three factors that underpin sustainable change are *focus, fit,* and *finish.*

Focus addresses the questions, What needs to be changed? and What is the best use of our human and capital resources at this time? The answers to these questions determine whether the change is being managed or not. Too often a problem arises and a "fix" is put in place without the necessary discussion of what is the best outcome in terms of the organization's vision. The short-sighted goal of "make this bad problem go away" many times takes precedence over "what is best for the organization in the long term?" Problems with a lot of "noise" associated with them (e.g., physician issues, legislative mandates, anything to do with the budget) create a great deal of organizational energy. However, it is absolutely critical that the amount of noise is not used to define the criticality of the need for change.

An all-too-common phenomenon that exists in today's healthcare is "the negative vortex of doom" (see Chapter 4). This is a workplace dominated by negativity. The most reinforced behaviors were those with the greatest negative and depressing elements. I call this dynamic *one-downsmanship*, the opposite of one-upsmanship.

Uncontrolled catharsis, negative energy, and toxic dumps have become *de rigueur* at many healthcare institutions without a clear focus. Dynamically what has occurred is that the organization's mission, values, vision, and strategy are so out of focus that they have lost their ability to direct behavior. In this absence of a clear focus, personal needs and expectations become the decision rules. The question changes from "What is best for the organization?" to "What is best for me?" Without a clear focus that transcends self-interest, it is impossible to manage change.

The right person must be fit into the right place at the right time with the right resources is a simple formula for success. Fit represents the second critical success element in any managed change process. Do they have the knowledge, skills, and capacity to complete the task? Do they want to do it—that is, Will they find meaning in the work? Will they be proud of their accomplishments? Titled executives can spend hours pondering the merits of financial investments. They may request several pro forma scenarios and return-on-investment projections. Yet when the time comes to make a decision about investing human capital, the decision may only take minutes or may even be delegated to a subordinate. Leaders understand that the human capital decision is at least as important as any financial decision. Leaders know that a "perfect" decision about a business venture can fail because the wrong person was selected to shepherd the change. On the other hand, a less-than-perfect business decision can be a wonderful success when managed by inspired followers.

Cecelia Wooden, ED.D., speaks often about how fit is a main determinant of retention of high performers in hospitals (Atchison and Wooden 2003). She states that the three main reasons staff leave hospitals are

1. their boss—people don't leave jobs, they leave their boss;
2. professional development—people leave when their professional skills are not developed; they "burn out"; and
3. values clash—people leave when their personal beliefs toward their profession and work run counter to the values that underpin the climate in their work environment.

The right personnel fit make the third managed change element relatively easy—finish. This sounds so simple—just finish the task; just get the change managed. However, the ability to finish can be a challenge. Hospitals are notorious for meetings, second guessing, and the (completely bogus) belief that a consensus is necessary for success. Two very powerful factors need to be in place to counteract healthcare's Pavlovian reflex to obfuscate a change process. First, the process must be guided by brutal metrics. Second, the finish must be crystallized with a celebration.

Brutal metrics are objective data sources that determine whether progress is being made. The absence of these unimpeachable milestones allows subjectivity, resistance, and even regression to seep into the change process. Hospitals obsess over the financial metrics. The brutality of these business measures ensure constant focus on the financial objectives with little room for variance. The same brutality must be in place for measures of change in the intangibles—for example, patient satisfaction, patient safety, and clinical quality. Without clear measures and targets, success (or failure) is impossible to measure. Without objective data, all humans default to subjectivity, characterized by rationalizations, excuses, and the preservation of the status quo. Measurement allows for the last (and often forgotten) step in a managed change process.

Celebration must be the last step in a managed change process. A formal party to mark the successful completion or an informal pat on the back to show the completion of an assignment represents the most important factor in reinforcing followers. They need the feedback for a job well done. Today's healthcare workplace seems to be driven by pressure to do more with less; the successful completion of one task is met with the immediate assignment of another. High performers are burdened with more work, with little time spent telling the high performers how valuable they are to corporate goals. Metaphorically, the process is like always inhaling; followers must exhale periodically. Celebrations give followers this opportunity. Kelly Mather has institutionalized celebration in her high-performance model—she calls it *fun*.

> "Warmth is a word that comes to mind in answer to what inspired followers. Simple behaviors like eye contact, finding out what their interests are, engaging them in decisions, and a sense of humor show people that your care."
>
> —*Donald Buckley*, PH.D., FACHE, *president and* CEO, *Chesapeake General Hospital, Chesapeake, Virginia*

Domain 5: The Vision

The corporate vision answers the two-part question, Where are we going, and how do we know we have arrived? Visions have three characteristics (they can have more, as long as these three are in place). The first, and most critical, characteristic of a vision is that it is inspirational; the second is that it must be directional; and the third is that it must be measurable. Without a vision that meets these three standards, people and organizations default to retrovisioning, defined earlier in the book as a situation in which, with no clear agreement on inspirational and measurable direction, the discussion focuses on the last big issue. Organizations without visions tend to be frozen in reactive, tactical response patterns. Such organizations are described as always in a crisis mode. Peter Senge (1990) did a wonderful job describing the importance of visions in his work *The Fifth Discipline:*

The Art and Practice of the Learning Organization. Collins and Porras (1994), in *Built to Last: Successful Habits of Visionary Companies,* makes a strong argument that visions are the essence of sustainable success.

A vision is an endgame. Visions drive *strategy,* strategy determines *tactics,* and tactics inform *individual performance.* Visions are states of being. When individuals make choices about behaviors that achieve the vision, their behavior increases the probability of success (Figure 10.3). For some unknown reason, titled executives say that visions are not possible in today's complicated and unpredictable healthcare world. Interestingly, these same individuals will spend hundreds of staff hours developing a budget, designing a building project, and calculating their personal retirement plan. Budgets, building, and retirement plans are *visions.* Each of these processes meets the three criteria for visions: inspirational (albeit inspiration from a potentially negative source in the case of the budget), directional, and measurable. The same mental and developmental processes used to develop these visions about the tangible elements of the organization can be used to create a vision about the intangibles. Titled executives might become excited about a new building, budget, or retirement option; however, followers only respond to visions about the intangibles. The best example of an inspirational vision is Martin Luther King Jr.'s statement, "I have a dream." Reverend King did not say, "I have a strategic plan!" His short statement was inspirational and directional and drove measurable steps to achievement. Effective visions can ignite followership—just like Reverend King's did.

Strategy follows the creation and communication of a vision. Henry Mintzberg (1994) wrote about the limits of strategic planning without an overriding vision. Visions are divided into strategic imperatives. These imperatives are implemented through tactical plans. Within each tactical plan there are specific accountabilities. The linear nature of moving from visions to individual

Figure 10.3: Chart of Transcendent Purpose

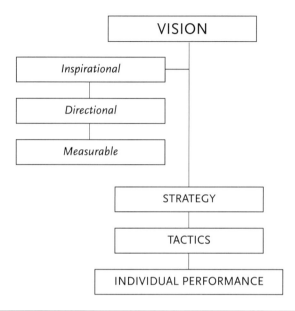

behavior ensures that followers know at each step their role and contribution for success.

Domain 6: The Corporate Values

Values define the way we do things—our *behavior*. The values are the most important variable in the long-term success of any enterprise. They identify not what you do, but how you do it. All airlines have very similar missions, visions, and business plans, so why is Southwest the only airline that has a consistent history of profitability? All discount retail merchants have the same goals, many even have the same type of structure and locations. Why is Wal-Mart the number one *Fortune* 500 company based on sales revenue and K-Mart has filed for bankruptcy? The answer lies in the underlying values that define the behavior of each employee. Southwest staff are followers of a few simple principles about how to behave with their customers.

"Sam's Way" is a mantra for everyone employed by Wal-Mart. Of course, Wal-Mart has sophisticated information and other business support systems. However, the consistently higher sales revenue and growth is driven by the millions of people who shop there because of the way they are treated. The corporate values must be meaningful—they cannot just be rhetoric used for marketing purposes. Lencioni's (2002) article, "Make Your Values Mean Something," supports the critical message of this chapter: Organizational success is always about the behavior of followers.

> "I see my role as the communicator, supporter, and cheerleader of our mission, values, and vision. My job is to inspire the marvelous people who work within this system and continue to do what it takes to get them pulling in the same direction."
>
> —Kevin Nolan, president and CEO, *Affinity Health System, Menasha, Wisconsin*

Ask this question as a quick test: Can you identify three behaviors that at least 80 percent of your employees display because they represent the corporate values? How about one behavior per value? If you want to see how far healthcare has drifted away from this essential and fundamental concept of values-based behavior, audit next Sunday's help-wanted ads. Take a look at how the ads are written for nurses. Are they promoting pay, benefits, and flexible work schedules, or are the ads focused on values such as quality, professionalism, partnerships with physicians, patient care, and customer satisfaction? My unscientific audits typically show a 10 to 1 ratio of pay to values. And we wonder why this industry is such a mess. We hire on the basis of the tangibles and get upset when the intangibles are terrible, resulting in yet another self-inflicted wound.

Understanding core values is easy. Watch how people make *decisions*. In an organization with a lot of followers, those followers' decisions will be based on the values of the organization. In an organization with titled executives who live only in the tangible business world, the staffs' decisions will be driven by personal values.

The last element of this domain is the *reward and recognition* system. A great deal of confusion continues to exist regarding the purpose and best methodology for effective reward and recognition. The article "Exposing the Myths of Employee Satisfaction" (Atchison 2003) discusses these concerns. The important lesson in terms of corporate values is to only reward those behaviors that are values driven and ignore or punish any behavior that run counter to the values. Reward and recognition programs that are not tied directly to values-based behaviors are more than useless. They are expensive and many times contradict the espoused reasons for such a program. Badly designed and implemented reward and recognition programs are another self-inflicted wound.

Domain 7: Employer of Choice

The number of followers is a good standard to use to determine if you are an employer of choice. Turnover rates, labor actions, employee and physician satisfaction data, pride indicators, ease of recruitment, strength of culture, and any other measurement of an intangible factor tells the degree to which your organization has a high or low potential for followers. Several books, articles, and seminars are available to help organizations become identified as the employer of choice. This chapter lists 21 followership variables in the seven major domains (triangles), introduced at the beginning of this chapter, that must be in place before the employer-of-choice designation can be made. An interesting report published by www.ctnet.com (2003) (Figure 10.1) supports the idea that the intangibles of the organization determine whether followers will choose to join it. It indicates that people work more for psychic income than financial income. Compensation only becomes the most important factor when the four more important factors do not exist in the workplace.

Table 10.1: Why People Decide to Quit

Responses given to the question, "Over the course of your career, what has been the most significant reason you have chosen to leave your employer?"

Lack of challenge and excitement	39%
Career path	27%
Corporate culture or value system	15%
Your boss	11%
Compensation	8%

Note: These results suggest that organizations looking to hold on to talented employees should concentrate on providing a stimulating work environment, not simply throw more money at workers.

Source: Christian & Timbers, www.ctnet.com. Used with permission.

Followers choose to work in an organization where they can be proud of their work, find joy in performing the day-to-day tasks, and are satisfied with the working conditions.

Pride is a seldom discussed but critically important element for followers. Pride typically results from the successful completion of a challenge or difficult task. Ask ten people where they find pride in their life. The answer will always contain some reference to being stretched beyond their perceived limits. Seldom will you hear talk about how proud they where that they lie in bed and watched TV all day. Such "lazy" behavior might make them satisfied (happy), but it will never make them proud. Employers of choice challenge their staff to higher performance.

Joy is, tragically, almost nonexistent in healthcare today. Joyful work is the highest level of adult behavior. Artists, athletes, parents, hobbyists, and others are able to find joy in the doing and pride in the outcome. Why has this wonderful human dynamic been eliminated from delivering care—one of the most noble professions? Healthcare as an industry is not the employer of choice, but, thankfully, there still exist several islands of healthcare professionals who follow their leaders because they exhibit all of the 21 FQ elements listed in this chapter. These rare organizations are the employers of choice mainly because the leaders have created an ecosystem in which pride, joy, and satisfaction thrive.

The continuums in Figures 10.4a–10.4h are measures of the 21 factors that are necessary to sustain followership. You may wish to assess yourself on these elements. You may also wish to use these continuums in a 360-degree-evaluation motif. Unlike many "leadership assessments," this survey can result in a negative score to reflect those titled executives who are destructive and even toxic. (Of course, they won't likely complete this survey.)

In Figure 10.4a, the first critical inputs to success are those personal traits of the leader. Courage, energy, and discipline

> "No matter what difficulties are currently confronting our organization, I try to always remember that I cannot put too much emphasis on the intangibles—they will either help us manage change or become a barrier to change."
>
> —*Raymond V. Ingham*, PH.D., FACHE, *president and CEO, Witham Health Services, Lebanon, Indiana*

underpin all future success. Figure 10.4b depicts the second step as a focus on the organization's mission, values, and vision. The leader helps to convert these words into focused behaviors. Figure 10.4c shows that high-performing leaders who create a positive corporate culture (ecosystem) produce followers. Leaders of strong cultures provide meaning, show respect, and allow staff to control the decisions that affect them. As shown in Figure 10.4d, followers understand why change must be made (to achieve the vision), they want the change to happen (to provide better services), and they control the change process. In Figure 10.4e, vision sets the direction and ignites the inspiration to move forward. Measuring vision achievement is the best way to manage sustainable change. For Figure 10.4f, values are the fuel that drive behavior. High-performing organizations have clear behaviors

Figure 10.4a: Followership Quotient—Leaders*

LEADERS:

The CEO of our organization . . .

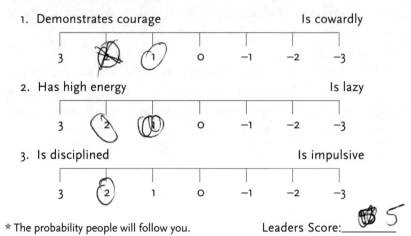

1. Demonstrates courage ———————————————— Is cowardly

   3   2   1   0   −1   −2   −3

2. Has high energy ———————————————— Is lazy

   3   2   1   0   −1   −2   −3

3. Is disciplined ———————————————— Is impulsive

   3   2   1   0   −1   −2   −3

* The probability people will follow you.   Leaders Score:_____ 5

Figure 10.4b: Followership Quotient—Corporate Culture*

CORPORATE CULTURE:

Our organization . . .

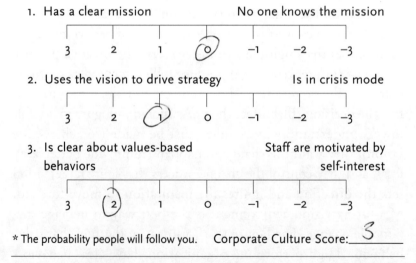

1. Has a clear mission ———— No one knows the mission

   3   2   1   0   −1   −2   −3

2. Uses the vision to drive strategy ———— Is in crisis mode

   3   2   1   0   −1   −2   −3

3. Is clear about values-based   Staff are motivated by
   behaviors   self-interest

   3   2   1   0   −1   −2   −3

* The probability people will follow you.   Corporate Culture Score:_3_____

Figure 10.4c: Followership Quotient—Followers*

FOLLOWERS:
Employees in our organization . . .

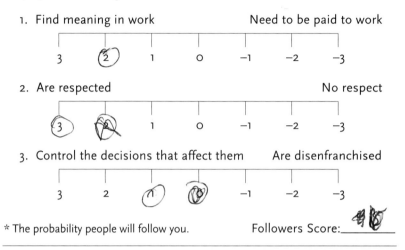

1. Find meaning in work   Need to be paid to work

    3   (2)   1   0   −1   −2   −3

2. Are respected   No respect

    (3)   (2)   1   0   −1   −2   −3

3. Control the decisions that affect them   Are disenfranchised

    3   2   (1)   (0)   −1   −2   −3

* The probability people will follow you.   Followers Score:_____

Figure 10.4d: Followership Quotient—Managing Change*

MANAGING CHANGE:
We move forward . . .

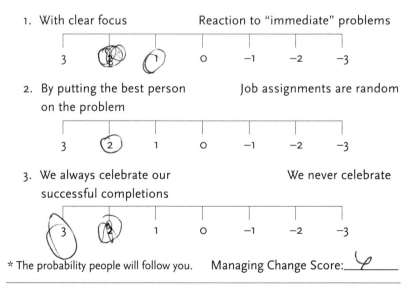

1. With clear focus   Reaction to "immediate" problems

    3   (2)   (1)   0   −1   −2   −3

2. By putting the best person   Job assignments are random
   on the problem

    3   (2)   1   0   −1   −2   −3

3. We always celebrate our   We never celebrate
   successful completions

    (3)   (2)   1   0   −1   −2   −3

* The probability people will follow you.   Managing Change Score:_____

Figure 10.4e: Followership Quotient—Vision*

VISION:
We use our vision . . .

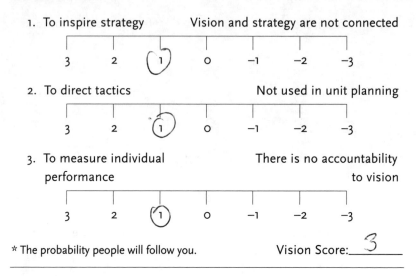

1. To inspire strategy   Vision and strategy are not connected

    3   2   (1)   0   −1   −2   −3

2. To direct tactics   Not used in unit planning

    3   2   (1)   0   −1   −2   −3

3. To measure individual   There is no accountability
   performance   to vision

    3   2   (1)   0   −1   −2   −3

* The probability people will follow you.   Vision Score: _3_

Figure 10.4f: Followership Quotient—Corporate Values*

CORPORATE VALUES:
Our core values . . .

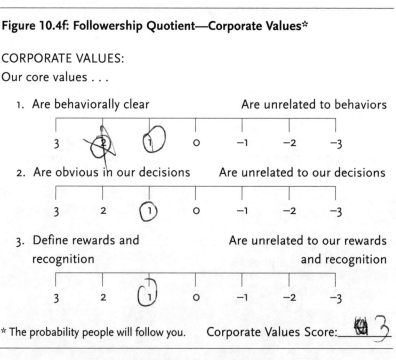

1. Are behaviorally clear   Are unrelated to behaviors

    3   (2)(1)   0   −1   −2   −3

2. Are obvious in our decisions   Are unrelated to our decisions

    3   2   (1)   0   −1   −2   −3

3. Define rewards and   Are unrelated to our rewards
   recognition   and recognition

    3   2   (1)   0   −1   −2   −3

* The probability people will follow you.   Corporate Values Score: _3_

Figure 10.4g: Followership Quotient—Employer of Choice*

EMPLOYER OF CHOICE:

The employees in our organization . . .

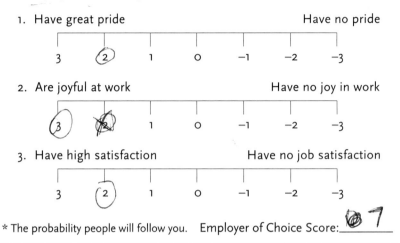

1. Have great pride   Have no pride

3   (2)   1   0   −1   −2   −3

2. Are joyful at work   Have no joy in work

(3)   2   1   0   −1   −2   −3

3. Have high satisfaction   Have no job satisfaction

3   (2)   1   0   −1   −2   −3

* The probability people will follow you.   Employer of Choice Score: _7_

Figure 10.4h: Followership Quotient—Total*

TOTAL FQ

Subscores:

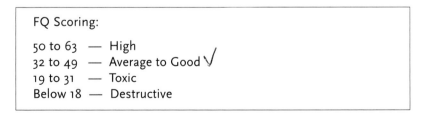

1. Leaders   5
2. Corporate Culture   8 · 2
3. Followers   4 · 0
4. Managing Change   0 ·
5. Vision   3 ·
6. Corporate Values   4 3
7. Employer of Choice   7
     Total   30 35

FQ Scoring:

50 to 63 — High
32 to 49 — Average to Good ✓
19 to 31 — Toxic
Below 18 — Destructive

that reflect their values. These behaviors are consistently displayed by all. Figure 10.4g supports the notion that leaders create an environment that attracts followers who manage change. This combination attracts high performers who continue the process of going from good to great. In Figure 10.4h, the score identifies the strengths and weaknesses in the organizational transformation process.

CONCLUSION

Followership is the critical factor in sustainable success of any organization. Many healthcare organizations have forgotten this truth. The external regulatory and internal staffing issues are just two of the pressures that will not go away. Titled executives, unfortunately, respond badly to these pressures and may even hurt the organization. Leaders know that their *only* job is to inspire followers who can thrive within these unpredictable but constant pressures. The cases and models presented in this book are examples of ways to return to a healthcare industry defined by leadership that focuses on the quality and spirit of the followers who provide great care to people in need.

REFERENCES

Atchison, T. 1990. "Turn Around, Leaders: Is Anyone Following?" *Hospitals* 64 (13): FB50, FB52.

———. 2002. "What Is Corporate Culture." *Trustee* 55 (4): 11.

———. 2003. "Exposing the Myths of Employee Satisfaction." *Healthcare Executive* 18 (3): 20–26.

Atchison, T., and J. S. Bujak. 2002. *Leading Transformational Change: The Physician-Executive Partnership*. Chicago: Health Administration Press.

Atchison, T., and C. K. Wooden. 2003. "Capitalize on Your Recruitment Investment: Building a Retention Culture." Seminar, June 11–12, Newport, RI. American College of Healthcare Executives.

Collins, J. 2001. *Good to Great: Why Some Companies Make the Leap . . . and Others Don't*. New York: HarperCollins.

Collins, J., and J. Porras. 1994. *Built to Last: Successful Habits of Visionary Companies*. New York: HarperCollins.

Dye, C. 2002. *Winning the Talent War: Effective Leadership in Healthcare*. Chicago: Health Administration Press.

Lencioni, P. 2002. "Make Your Values Mean Something." *Harvard Business Review* 80 (7): 113–17.

Mintzberg, H. 1994. "The Fall and Rise of Strategic Planning." *Harvard Business Review* (Jan/Feb): 107–14.

Senge, P. 1990. *The Fifth Discipline: The Art and Practice of the Learning Organization*. New York: Currency/Doubleday.

Wheatley, M. 1999. *Leadership and the New Science*. San Francisco: Berret-Koehler Publishing.

Epilog

THE BOOK HAS ended; another journey is complete. Any frustrations that occurred during the writing of this book were a small price to pay for the pleasure of working with the people about whom this book is written. The interviews and associations with those healthcare leaders who have many followers was truly a joy. These exceptional people seem to live only to create and maintain an environment that allows individuals to make a difference. They are healthcare's chief leadership officers. Regardless of age, gender, years of experience, academic credentials, military or civilian status, or location, these special individuals all possess the five characteristics that inspire followers:

1. Competence
2. Integrity
3. Consistency
4. Courage
5. Humility

The two most important findings of this book are that (1) these five characteristics must be in place to inspire followers and

(2) all five must exist. You cannot have four out of five; you can not be an 80 percent leader.

The sadness in writing this book came from the realization that a large group of healthcare executives seem to live only to create an environment that ensures self-preservation. These are the titled executives who at best do not hurt anyone and who at worst are so self-absorbed that they create toxic work environments. An executive title without followers has an illusion of power. These titled executives create a workplace without a soul.

Skills, knowledge, and techniques are important, but they are the tools of the craft. Without a constant focus on "making good better for all," there is no joy, no pride, no elevation above the need to survive—there are no followers. Chief leadership officers take their craft to the level of an art. Schools and continuing education teach the tools, but they do not teach soul.

About the Author

TOM ATCHISON, ED.D., is president and founder of The Atchison Consulting Group, Inc. Since 1984, Dr. Atchison has consulted with healthcare organizations on managed change programs, team building, and leadership development. He also has consulted to the military, healthcare vendors, and government agencies on the intangible aspects of healthcare.

His consulting practice focuses on measuring and managing the intangibles that drive change. Typically, he consults to senior executives, managers, trustees, and physician leaders.

Dr. Atchison gives presentations to thousands of healthcare professionals a year on the elements of effective organizations. He has written and been featured in a number of articles and audio and video tapes about motivation, managed change, team building, and leadership. He is the author of *Turning Healthcare Leadership Around* and coauthor with Joseph S. Bujak, M.D., of *Leading Transformational Change: The Physician-Executive Partnership.*

Dr. Atchison's expertise in healthcare is built on more than 30 years' experience in a variety of management positions in healthcare institutions and organizations. Dr. Atchison is a member of the American College of Healthcare Executives. He earned his doctoral degree in human resource development from Loyola University of Chicago.